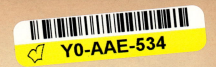

INTIMATE REVELATIONS AND
KNOWLEDGEABLE ADVICE NEVER STOP
COMING—IN THE BOOK THAT KEEPS
GOING WHEN ALL OTHERS LEAVE OFF!

The men and women interviewed in this book
had to fulfill two requirements.

They had to be eminent in the area of sex, either
in their professional work or their legendary
private lives. And they had to agree to hold
nothing back.

**If you wonder about any and every area of male
sexual performance in theory and in practice . . .
if you want to know exactly what turns women
on . . . if you'd like to learn the kind of lover
the new breed of liberated lady is looking for . . .
if you're curious about the part that sex actually
plays in the world of the beautiful people . . . this
is your chance to truly find out—**

WHAT MAKES A MAN G.I.B.*
*good in bed

Books of Special Interest from SIGNET

What Makes a Man G.I.B.*

*good in bed

by Wendy Leigh

Afterword from Gore Vidal

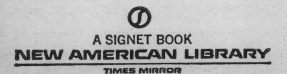

A SIGNET BOOK

NEW AMERICAN LIBRARY

TIMES MIRROR

For Kevin Maitland, who helped me every slow page.

Copyright © 1979 by Wendy Leigh

SIGNET TRADEMARK REG. U.S. PAT. OFF. AND FOREIGN COUNTRIES
REGISTERED TRADEMARK—MARCA REGISTRADA
HECHO EN CHICAGO, U.S.A.

SIGNET, SIGNET CLASSICS, MENTOR, PLUME AND MERIDIAN BOOKS
are published by The New American Library, Inc.,
1301 Avenue of the Americas, New York, New York 10019

FIRST PRINTING, NOVEMBER, 1979

1 2 3 4 5 6 7 8 9

PRINTED IN THE UNITED STATES OF AMERICA

DEDICATION

This book is for Zsa Zsa Gabor, who suggested
America in the first place.

For Irving Mansfield, who helped me survive the
low points.

For Russ Gallen, Scott Meredith and Jonathan Clowes,
with thanks for the high points.

And especially for Carolyn Stromberg, who believed
in me through it all.

ACKNOWLEDGMENTS

I should like to thank Domenica Fitzgerald in Los Angeles, Margot and George Comley in San Francisco, Eric Drache in Las Vegas, Ann Drache in New Jersey, and Dorette Luedecke and Filou in New York for their invaluable hospitality and warmth.

I am very thankful to Patrick Lichfield, Oscar Abolafia, and Lorenz Zatecky for their photographs; to Barbara Daly for her makeup; Keith at Smile, London, and Jerry Brennan at Vidal Sassoon, New York, for hair; Spaghetti of London, Annie Gough at Gemini, and Rizkallah of New York for their clothes. To the Inlingua Language School, Konstanz, for their translations of the Italian and French interviews. To Rebecca Michael and Martha Nelson for their secretarial assistance.

I received introductions and help in arranging interviews from many people, I should like to thank them all—especially Sherry Grant and Jerry Pam in Los Angeles. Diana Stammers, Alan Markfield, Wayne Darwen, Roz Starr, Carmen Lavia, Frederick Davies, the Contessa Christina Paolozzi Bellin, Joan Sands, and Gus Ober in New York. Yvonne DeValera, Peter Noble, Elena Overs, and Paul Callan in London, and John Penrose in Rome. With special thanks to Susan Lamb, who promoted "Speaking Frankly" to perfection.

CONTENTS

PART III: THE FEMALE CELEBRITIES   127

INTRODUCTION

The title of this book is only one of many questions I posed when interviewing a galaxy of celebrities, psychologists, sociologists, and superstuds. The book not only presents a kaleidoscope of answers to that title question but also investigates contemporary attitudes to love, sex, and relationships.

The book could be labeled a celebrity book, a confessional book, or a how-to sex book. I prefer to dispense with labels and quote instead Gore Vidal's comment: "Any exploration of the extraordinary variety of human sexual response acts like those funhouse mirrors in showing us as we really are. And even though they may distort and mock the human figure, they never cease to reveal the real thing."

The faces reflected in this particular mirror are the faces of some of America's most famous men and women. Their attitudes run the gamut from conventional to progressive, from romantic to permissive, and the spotlight is always on the individual—never on the statistic.

Interviewee Selection

I have explained my reasons for interviewing experts and superstuds in the revelant sections of the book. I decided to interview celebrities because I wanted to talk to visible, identifiable people. I hoped to replace the clinical anonymity of sex surveys and the gynecological exaggerations of sex magazines with recognizable individuals seriously discussing their desires and attitudes to love, sex, and relationships.

The celebrities spoke to me with surprising frankness, refusing to project themselves as supermen or superwomen. Ultimately everyone can compare notes with the celebrities and somewhere find viewpoints, problems, and desires similar to his or her own.

Interviewing Technique

I learned about interviewing through working in British TV and radio. At the age of twenty-one I was fired from my first job—researching an ITV boat program—because the producer discovered I couldn't swim. Surviving, I went on to work for BBC TV and radio as an investigative reporter. Some of my most adventurous projects included investigating fraudulent model agencies by posing as an aspiring model, working as a door-to-door salesgirl aiding cameramen to infiltrate an illegal sales team, and traveling from London to Paris with forty-five pregnant French girls for a program exposing abortion "package tours" that subjected clients to inhumane conditions. I also interviewed celebrities for BBC radio, and during an interview, Zsa Zsa Gabor suggested that I try to work in America. I took her advice.

When I started interviewing for my first book in America, I realized that I had to discard British television's cardinal rule about interviewing celebrities: "Research, research, research—know every fact about your interviewee before you meet them." That same rule operates in the American media, but with my project I got better results if I reversed all rules and *forgot* every fact about a celebrity, because every fact led to asking all the questions that every other journalist had asked—questions not necessarily revelant to my project. Instead I found that if I interviewed without a list of facts or expectations, the interview would flow more naturally. So I always avoided trying to elicit any specific responses suggested to me by a celebrity's press cuttings. The questions varied from interview to interview. At the beginning of each section of the book I have listed the questions I asked in that particular section. Some of the interviews are set out in question-and-answer format in order to highlight the variety of topics covered in that interview. Each individual celebrity interview begins with an introduction explaining why I interviewed that particular celebrity, how I arranged the interview, where I conducted the interview, how the celebrity treated me, how I reacted to them, and how the reality of the person conflicted with or corresponded to their public image.

Each interview was conducted on tape (I still have the tapes), and if a remark was made by an interviewee off tape it was not included in the book. After the interview I transcribed the tape and rearranged the order of the material (in the interests of fluency), but didn't radically alter anything. Every interviewee in the book was required to sign a release and was given the right to approve, change, or cut his or her own interview.

Themes and Topics

The title topic—What Makes a Man Good in Bed—is dealt with by most of the interviewees, and each section in the book ends with a summary of the conclusions reached by the interviewees in that section. The summaries deal with the title question—but the book is rich in other themes. Below are some of them.

Sex in America in the Past

As Letitia Baldrige (Amy Vanderbilt) says, "In the old days a woman would never talk about sex"—and this book would certainly have never been written. The openness of celebrities when discussing sex is very much a product of the sexual revolution—and so am I. Even fifteen years ago, any woman interviewing on the subject of love and sex would not have been received as a legitimate journalist. The fact that I and my subject were always treated with respect is symptomatic of dramatic changes in attitudes toward women and sex. Nevertheless, my interviewees still voice nostalgia for the past—for the days when women were still afraid of pregnancy and of disgracing their families and were told that no decent woman was capable of feeling passion. Female interviewees talk about the death of romance, "necking," and the now almost-obsolete dating game. Many male interviewees recall their teenage boasts of nonexistent sexual conquests, visits to $5 brothels, and '50s "scoring."

Sex in the Present

The book centers on today's different love styles. Experts talk about myths of the '70s, the lack of a moral structure, men going to bed with women indiscriminately, and both men and women measuring themselves by media standards and feeling inadequate. Male interviewees criticize sex in the present; people have too few worries nowadays so instead they worry about sex, girls throw themselves around communes, and men become impotent because they feel obliged to be good lovers. Female interviewees talk about male stress, say they find it easier to have sex nowadays and that today people talk about sex more—and do it less.

The First Time

They say you never forget the first time. I lost my virginity three weeks before my twentieth birthday. The man was English, an executive for a Middle Eastern advertising company, and had invited me to go to Beirut with him. Before Beirut, I decided that the time was ripe (and so was I) to "lose" my virginity. So instead of Beirut, I found myself in a flat in Bournemouth (a respectable English seaside resort). The sex was more satisfying than I had ever imagined—but afterward I cooked breakfast, burned the bacon, had a fight with the man, and refused to go to Beirut with him. Nonetheless, my virginity was "lost" in true 1970s style—without guilt or wedding ring. Since I "lost" my virginity, I have never switched roles and "found" a man's virginity, or lusted after any teenagers. So I was amazed when seven male interviewees confessed to me that their virginity had been "taken" from them when they were only in their early teens.

The Relationship Between Love and Sex

My mother says, "Bad sex ruins a love relationship, but good sex doesn't necessarily make one." Whereas *I* sometimes say, "Bad love relationships often ruin good sex"—because I don't feel that love and sex *must* always be related. I agree with a comment made to me by literary critic Kenneth Tynan: "People who say you've got to have sex *with* love are like people who say you must only travel by Concorde." Most of my interviewees say that sex with love is the ideal. Male interviewees say that sex with love is rare, that curiosity has put more people into bed than romance, and that a man should *think* he is in love with every woman with whom he goes to bed. Female interviewees say that they are incapable of having sex without love, that love detracts from wildness, that you can't separate sex from the rest of a relationship, and that attraction is more important than love.

Attitudes Toward Woman's Liberation

As a career woman I feel that my professional status is a product of my liberation. Both my mother and my grandmother were liberated businesswomen, and I grew up automatically expecting equality and independence. I believe in woman's liberation and live it, but continually encounter men who don't. I think the book indicates the ever-present gap between woman's liberation in theory, and woman's liberation as lived (or not lived).

The experts talk about the effect of woman's liberation on men (both negative and positive); they say that men want assertive women, that men are disturbed because women no longer cater to their archaic "courtship" routines, and that men no longer feel so virile because women are now financially independent. Male interviewees say that woman's liberation hasn't changed the relationship between men and women, that women are no longer seduced by cliched approaches, that men become impotent because of women's liberation, and that liberated women are usually very feminine. Female interviewees say that women's liberation has not altered relationships between men and women, and that it will take ten to fifteen years for the women's movement to have an effect.

Sex Related to Fame and Profession

Many interviewees discuss the relationship between sex and profession, and the effect of fame on their relationships with the opposite sex. Male interviewees comment on sex and the powerful man, sex and artists, sex and sportsmen, sex with groupies, sex and being a sex symbol. Female interviewees talk about male sex symbols, having sex with a famous lover, feeling pressured to live up to a "sexy" image, and the problems of deciding whether a man wants them for themselves for for their image.

In the past three years I have found myself in similar situations. I've interviewed insecure male stars terrified of rejection, I've met superstuds set on proving themselves sexually, and I've had relationships with powerful men who were unable to switch off the power. My books sometimes transform me into a red rag to men who think they are bulls—so that like Carroll Baker, I've met men who imagined my "sexpertise" would solve their problems, and like Debbie Harry I've sometimes felt obliged to act the role of "sex symbol."

How to Approach a Woman

Men I interviewed repeatedly expressed the discomfort they feel when approaching a woman. Traditional male fears of rejection have been intensified by the sexual revolution. Fifteen years ago if a woman refused to go to bed with a man, he could (rightly or wrongly) attribute her refusal to the woman's virginity or her fear of pregnancy. In the permissive "yes years" of the '70s and '80s, a woman's refusal to go to bed with a man amounts to a stark personal rejection. Fear of that very personal type of rejection often causes men to be clumsy when approaching a woman.

Women I interviewed agreed with me about cliché'd, unimaginative male approaches. Most of us had encountered the crudest approaches in Hollywood (first date: "Are you going to bed with me before dinner or after?"). I am not suggesting that men must always make the first approach—but while they predominantly do, I think many men ought to learn how.

My questions were designed to explore the many schools of thought (or lack of thought) on how to approach a woman. The experts advise good manners, making an inoffensive gesture (like touching a woman's hand), not propositioning a woman unless you are certain she is very receptive, not using lines published in *Playboy* fifteen years ago, not going to bed with every woman just because she is available.

Male interviewees talk about their tips for pre-bed approaches to women. Don't ask a woman verbally—just exchange looks. Tell every woman that she is beautiful, wait till you feel the electricity flow between you, look into a woman's eyes and judge the extent of her attraction to you, be honest with a woman. Female interviewees talk about male approaches they dislike; too many clichés, lines like "Hey babe—let's go to bed," and insincere offers of a "meaningful relationship." Approaches they like: wooing and flowers, flattery and softness, friendship and kindness.

How to Find Out What A Woman Wants and Fantasizes

The book emphasizes techniques of sexual communication, clues and ways to find out what a woman wants sexually. The experts agree that many people still circle one another sexually and are often unwilling to reveal their fantasies and desires for fear of rejection or shocking their partner.

I think women need more help than men in expressing their sexual desires. No man has ever told me that he was afraid to ask for what he wanted in bed—only that a woman had refused to do it. It is still accepted that a man is entitled to make sexual demands. If a man is unwilling to make certain demands on someone he loves, the outlet of prostitution is always available to satisfy any "perversions." Most women are unable to use that same outlet, to make sexual requests easily, or to reveal their fantasies openly. Thus the man who enables a woman to reveal her fantasies and desires may unleash years of sexual repression, and may satisfy that woman more fully than any previous partner. Therefore many of my questions are aimed at exploring ways of sexual communication, and techniques by which a man can discover what the woman with whom he is involved really wants.

The experts suggest ways in which men can recognize specific types of women, prescribe verbal techniques designed to reveal a woman's desires, and give advice on the right time, place, and way of finding out a woman's fantasies. The male interviewees echo and contradict the experts' advice, and the female interviewees discuss whether or not a man should literally *ask* a woman what she likes.

Sex in the Future

Most of the interviewees in the book discuss sexual omens for the 1980s—the quality of love, sex, and relationships they believe their children should inherit.

About the Author

I went to America to write this book and live out all my media-induced romantic fantasies of America. Growing up in the TV age, my generation was subjected to a barrage of American movies and television shows: *77 Sunset Strip, Viva Las Vegas, Hollywood Hotel, Sunset Boulevard*. And just as American tourists want to visit British historical monuments, I wanted to visit American movie locations. So when I picked my first American hotel I chose the location of a movie I'd never seen—*42nd Street*. I stayed in my first American hotel right there on 42nd Street—and spent my first American night wondering why American hotel walls were so thin, and why American men were so vulgar.

The next day I flew to California, armed with tape recorder, $400, and assignments from British newspapers and magazines, which all wanted interviews with

Robert Redford and Paul Newman. My aim was to write my first two books, which I believed in, and I assumed that the fat fees promised for my Newman and Redford interviews would support me until the books were written. After two weeks as a total stranger in Los Angeles, with little money, no driver's license, and no work permit, I realized that Newman and Redford were shatteringly remote—and that my fantasies of California really *were* fantasies. The reality was totally without romance.

My impression was reinforced by various offers designed to upgrade my financial status. A graying Persian millionaire, with a green Rolls-Royce, offered me my own apartment in exchange for monthly "scenes" with his seventeen-year-old Mexican girlfriend (who wore white lipstick and drank strawberry-flavored champagne). A Beverly Hills business manager offered me $400 a month, provided I agree to entertain him every Friday, in his room at the Beverly Wilshire Hotel (where, if necessary, he could take urgent business calls). And a Las Vegas cab driver ("on behalf of a major hotel") offered me $500 "a time" to cater to the whims of VIP gamblers. All three offers were refused in true Doris Day style, and I remained a struggling but virtuous Hollywood heroine.

Eventually I found more legitimate employment and investigated pregnancy-testing clinics for a national newspaper, researched a BBC TV documentary on Charles Manson, and spent two and a half days on the telephone trying to sell Bicentennial pens to undertakers. I rapidly became aware that far from starring in *That's Entertainment* I was, in fact, merely an extra trapped on the set of *Day of the Locust*.

Comparatively undaunted, I started the book, often spending my days interviewing in opulent Beverly Hills homes far removed from my own. During fifteen months in California I lived in six different apartments and learned all about the Hollywood sleaze which exists close to the Beverly Hills glamour. First I lived in a

Sunset Strip rooming house which was aptly nicknamed "The Beginning and the End"—because you either began there with no money or ended there with no money. My second address seemed far more comfortable, until there was a burglary during which only two things were stolen: the landlady's daughter's pot, and my tape recorder. Next I house-sat for two lesbians (then meditating in Big Sur), fed their goldfish ("Light and Dark"), and avoided unannounced visits from the Buddhist next door (reputedly a relative of the Hearsts).

Then I lived in the wing of a luxury Bel Air residence where the landlady, a Scarsdale import (stamped with Gucci, Cardin, and Louis Vuitton) complete with sculptured plaster nails and an EST diploma, mitigated my poverty with pearls dropped directly from Werner's million-dollar lips ("What is, is"). After the lady "experienced" that I didn't know (or want to go) where she was "coming from," I moved out. A friend offered me her floor—I accepted—and I spent two days frostily sleeping on the floor of an up-market Malibu nudist camp. In desperation I rented a Hollywood apartment, sight unseen. The "furnished apartment" on Poinsettia Street turned out to be just one room, with no windows, no furniture—just a mattress, with fleas on the floor and mouse droppings behind the drapes. Hooray for Hollywood.

Finally after a few celebrity interviews I went back to New York and discovered that I did like New York in June, even in a $40-a-week hotel with no air conditioning. In New York I met Irving Mansfield, Jacqueline Susann's widower, who encouraged me to struggle on with my project, presenting me with a copy of *Valley of the Dolls* inscribed: "This book was the biggest fiction best seller of all time. She only got a $1,000 advance—so you see—there is always hope." I began to believe there was. I borrowed money from friends, worked hard on the book, and never forgot psychic Sybil Leek's premonition that my books would be successful.

Less than a year after the Poinsettia Hollywood "apartment," I drove past it in a limousine (with a color TV in it) on my way to appear on *The Tomorrow Show*. My books were a success, and my experiences surviving Hollywood horrors even became a major discussion point with celebrities who had also survived similar squalor. Today I travel all over the world (still avoiding Hollywood if possible). I've talked on the most intimate level with the most incredible people—with dukes, duchesses, superstars, men whose pictures I worshiped when I was ten, and women whose films contributed to the romantic fantasies which first brought me to America.

I have lived out all those romantic fantasies. I've breakfasted by the shores of the Caribbean, lunched in Las Vegas, had cocktails in Palm Springs, dined in Rome, and danced till dawn at Studio 54 in New York and Regine's in Paris. I've been wooed by dazzling men in surroundings of unbelievable glamour. But I've also learned that you don't always find romance in a luxury hotel suite or on a tropical island—and that romance is equally likely to be found in one room in the back streets of New York.

The books have not only altered my attitude to romance, they have also altered my attitude to sex. I have learned that sexual desires are as individual as fingerprints and that everyone should try to be true to his or her own "fingerprint" and allow a partner to be true to his or her own. There are no formulas for sexual happiness; there are no instant clues to success in relationships. Only individuals. This book has tried to mirror the desires, the quality, and the uniqueness of some of them.

Part I

The Experts

The aim of this section is to define male sexual problems and the difficulties suffered by men in communicating sexually; to discuss the effects of woman's sexual liberation on men and what women today want from men sexually; and to provide expert advice to men. Apart from those themes the experts explore a myriad of topics related to men, male sexuality, and male/female relationships.

Interviewees Selected and Topics Discussed

I first talked to Dr. Wardell Pomeroy, co-author of The Kinsey Reports, because I wanted him to briefly summarize male sexual problems past and present. Then to Dr. Martin Cole, sex educationalist, on all areas of male sexual and courtship education, and to Dr. Emerson Symonds, sex-surrogate trainer, on male sexual problems communicated via feedback from trained surrogates, and to Pauline Abrams, sex therapist, on how male sexual problems can be cured. Moving from the physical, I talked to psychologist Dr. James Hemming on male trends and problems in courtship and communication. The previous experts repeatedly debated whether or not the women's liberation movement has had negative effects on male sexuality, so I talked to leading feminist Kate Lloyd, who, through her magazine, *Working Woman*, receives regular feedback on how both men and women are coping with women's lib. Then I talked to Dr. Herb Goldberg, male liberationist and psychoanalyst, on the problems and rewards men experience when dealing with the liberated woman. Next I talked to social arbitrator Letitia Baldrige on the new male sexual etiquette. I finished by interviewing psychoanalyst Dr. Erika Padan Freeman on male psychology and behavior and on omens for male sexuality in the '70s.

Questions Posed to the Experts

My questions were designed to elicit facts on men for themselves and for women who care about men. I wanted to test current theories on male sexuality and find out what men want out of sex, what women want from men, and how experts can help men sexually. These are the questions I asked.

Has today's sexual climate created specific problems for men?

What is the effect of the commercialization of sex on men?

How are male sexual problems related to age?

How are male psychological problems in dealing with women age-related?

What kinds of sexual education do men need?

How do you measure male sex drive?

How does a man learn to have sex?

Do teenagers still exaggerate their sexual experiences?

What kind of problems do men have in a pre-bed situation?

How should a man proposition a woman?

When should a man proposition a woman?

How are men affected when a woman rejects their advances?

How should a man cope with the advances of a woman?

Is there a great difference between male and female courtship behavior?

What problems do men face the first time they go to bed with a new woman?

How can a man judge in advance what kind of woman he is going to bed with?

How can a man discover what a woman wants sexually?

How can a man communicate what he wants sexually?

Should a man stick to a sexual routine?

How do you define male sexual goals?

How do men rate themselves sexually?

Is it normal for a man to occasionally fail sexually?

Can a woman help a man who is impotent?

How can the premature ejaculator be helped?

Do men still worry about penis size?

Do men with large penises have more sexual self-confidence or less?

Is it important for a man to give a woman oral sex?

How should a man give a woman oral sex?

Are men under more or less pressure to perform sexually nowadays?

What kinds of sexual situations create performance pressure?

How are men reacting to female sexual liberation?

Is the liberated woman causing impotence?

Has female sexual liberation caused any problems for men?

Does a "new woman" exist who is rating men sexually?

Have men anything to fear sexually from the new woman?

How would you advise the older man to cope with the liberated woman?

What do you think women want from men sexually?

What are the differences in male and female sexual enjoyment?

Do men think it is important to love the woman they are in bed with?

Is there a new sexual etiquette for men?

How are sexuality and profession related?

Can you describe the macho man?

Can you profile the powerful man sexually?

Can you profile the sadistic man sexually?

Can you profile the masochistic man sexually?

Can you profile the liberated man sexually?

What advice would you give a man who wants to be good in bed in a woman's judgment?

The experts shatter clichés, present facts, and summarize their findings in all fields related to male sexuality. The experts not only inform, but also advise, and provide a basis to the book from which men and women can compare their sexual experiences, thoughts, and feelings.

Dr. Wardell Pomeroy: On Male Sexuality Since Kinsey

The Kinsey Report on male sexuality published in 1948 was the first comprehensive study of male sexuality. I interviewed its co-author, Dr. Wardell Pomeroy, for an expert's view of traditional and current male sexual problems and myths. The interview, brief and to the point, also crystallizes and comments on some of the book's many themes: difficulties encountered in sexual communication, the effect of women's liberation on men, what women want sexually, and advice to men. I started the interview by asking Dr. Pomeroy how the world has changed sexually for men since the publication of the Kinsey Reports.

Men today face the same problems as they did when we published the Kinsey Reports: the inability to express feelings and desires, inadequacy in interpreting female sexuality, and, in general, a lack of communication. Even though today's popular press is more open about sex, people are not open to one another in their personal lives.

Has today's sexual climate created any additional problems?

Yes. New sexual myths have developed in the 1970s. First, there is the myth that sexual problems can be cured very easily through the work of people like Masters and Johnson. We find that while lesser sexual problems are quickly cured, the more difficult ones are not. There is also the myth that simultaneous orgasms are best for a couple—when they in reality are often not. Then there is the myth that penis size is absolutely irrelevant to the sexual satisfaction of a woman—which is an extreme reaction to the old myth that penis size was vital. There is also the myth that sexual technique is more important than the relationship.

Has female sexual liberation created any problems for men?

Currently there is a big argument as to whether men are threatened by female liberation, and whether it has resulted in men becoming impotent and feeling inadequate about their sexual abilities. I believe that argument is invalid, because in my experience, men *want* women to be more assertive and expressive of their sexual desires.

What do you think women want men to be sexually?

I think women want men to be tender, concerned, and sensitive to their feelings. They want a man who is not in a hurry and who enjoys the *process* of sex. One of the major differences between men and women is that the process of sex is terribly important to women—they are interested in the journey and not in the end result—whereas men are very sexually goal-oriented.

How would you define the sexual goals of the male?

Erection, penetration, and ejaculation. The male enjoys results and not the process. He rates himself on the basis of his performance—the size of his penis, how long he lasts, how many orgasms he has, and how many times he makes the woman come.

What is your advice to the man who wants to be good in bed for a woman?

To concentrate on his feelings and the woman's. To remember that sex doesn't have to be verbal communication—but that it can also be body communication. To listen to a woman's body, her words and her silences. Not to be in a hurry—but to revel in the moment and not look for anything else beyond.

Dr. Martin Cole:
On Male Sexual Myths

Dr. Martin Cole is director of the Institute of Sex Education and Research, Birmingham, England. I was surprised to discover that some men still need sex education and wanted to ask Dr. Cole about the kinds of men who consult him. I also talked to him about how men exaggerate their prowess, the problems men have when approaching a woman, and the difficulties men face the first time they go to bed with a new woman, and I asked him for his general advice to men. I ended the interview feeling depressed by Dr. Cole's verdict that what women want from men is impossible. I started the interview by referring to Wardell Pomeroy's sexual myths of the '70s and asked Dr. Cole how these myths had developed.

Myths develop about male sexuality because men continually misrepresent themselves sexually. They exaggerate their prowess, and never report the truth about what they really do in bed. Women boast about their husbands' sexual performance, and men tell locker-room stories—so that male sexuality is forever under scrutiny. False standards develop and men become sexually insecure because they are afraid that every other man is doing something better in bed.

What kind of men need sexual education?

I've seen men of thirty who were astounded to discover you could have intercourse in more than one position. I see other men with low sex drives who just opt out of sex because that is easier. They may have girlfriends, but they don't really care about them sexually. A man's sex drive can be partially measured by masturbation. A man in his twenties who masturbates once a day is regarded as having an average sex drive. Whereas a man in his twenties who masturbates less than once a month would be regarded as having a fairly low sex drive. However, ninety percent of the men I see with sex problems, DO have a fairly high sex drive, but have been brought up in a restrictive way, which has caused conflict and made them sexually anxious. Other men I see are inadequately programmed to have sex—guilt and anxiety have made them deny their sexual feelings, so that they have sexual stagefright and can't operate at all.

What kind of problems do men encounter before they go to bed with a woman?

Approaching a woman can be difficult, and men often have a great problem in integrating sex with relationships. There are some men who feel that sex has nothing to do with relationships—to them sex is a burden to be offloaded quickly, with minimum expense. Those men usually end up with prostitutes, because a relationship with a prostitute is transient, contractual, and therefore the man can opt out whenever he likes. Men who *are* able to have sex in the context of a relationship also often have blocks in courtship behavior which lead to a buildup of anxiety before bed. I would never advise a man to make a verbal approach to a woman—because it is very difficult to *ask* a woman to go to bed in a way that is both sensitive and inviting. I think a man should approach a woman nonverbally, with a physical gesture that is nonsexual—like touching the woman's hand. If a man has spent two or three hours with a woman and still is not sure if she wants to go to bed with him, he shouldn't push. A man should never go to bed with a woman unless he is absolutely sure of her. Men today are often very like sexual scavengers—they go to bed indiscriminately—and unless a man is a stallion he is a fool to go to bed with the wrong girl, because if he does he will make a mess of it.

What problems do men face sexually the first time they go to bed with a new woman?

The first time can be nerve-racking for a man, if he has failed before in a first-time situation. This creates a vicious circle of fear of failure and failure of fear. Loss of erection is always extremely threatening for a man, because he gets immediate feedback. The woman might say she doesn't mind—but the man will only interpret that as patronizing. The best way a woman can help a

man who is impotent is not to say a word, because
nothing verbal can help a man who has failed in bed.
In any case, every man should remember that most
men fail sexually now and again; you can be distracted
by worries, you can be frightened, or have drunk too
much. None of that means you have a sexual problem.
Men are often afraid of not living up to some indefin-
able expectation that no one has ever articulated. Patient after patient has come to me complaining that he
can't make love for very long—"only three-quarters of
an hour." Which is actually good—if the man is going
for all that time. The only research on the subject says
ninety percent of men will ejaculate before half an
hour. Sexuality is also age-related; a twenty-five-year-
old man ejaculates an average of three or four times a
night, but a man in his forties should not be disappointed if he has only one ejaculation a night. Men often expect too much of themselves.

*What do you think women really expect and want
from a man?*

Women want the impossible. They want a man who
is sensitive, who has a feminine streak, so that he is
perceptive, aware, and to whom they can talk. But they
also want a man who is an assertive, strong, and sexual
animal. Women want to feel secure and loved within a
relationship, but they also want to be fucked. A
woman wants to be loved one moment and raped the
next. Men are more deficient in the first than in the
second; they are probably better at fucking than at
building up an emotional, sensitive relationship.

*What advice would you give to a man who wants
to be good in bed for a woman?*

Try to recognize the type of woman you are in bed
with. A sensible man goes to bed only with his type of
woman and also realizes that not every woman is going

to be good for him. Once in bed with the woman a man should try to discover the sort of woman she is. The first time a man goes to bed with a woman he should talk fantasies to her—describe a series, and ask the woman which one she prefers. That will indicate her type. There is a sexual typology of women. A very sexual woman is aroused by only a touch and doesn't need the paraphernalia of fantasies. Whereas a masochistic woman tends to be fairly unresponsive, is unable to form a lasting relationship, and never gets orgasms through intercourse. She has rape fantasies, wants to be brutalized until she can't think anymore, and is only satisfied sexually when she is dominated. The very orgasmic woman gets full pelvic orgasms quickly, and is not promiscuous, because she is happy. But whatever type of woman he is in bed with, a man should remember to treat her like a human being and not a sex object. Try to communicate with her as an equal with all the sensitivity he possesses. And every man should remember that just as a woman should always try to be both prostitute and princess, a man should try to be both a Casanova and a prince.

Emerson Symonds:
On Male Sexual Problems

Emerson Symonds runs the Sensory Awareness Center in San Bernardino, California, where he trains both men and women to be sex surrogates. The process by which he trains them is not relevant to this book, so I haven't dealt with it. Instead I interviewed Emerson Symonds about the feedback he has received from surrogates regarding male sexual problems. He also talked to me about how boys bluff their way through sex, how men need to forget sex manuals, how men stick to old sexual routines and are unable to cope with women who no longer accept those routines, how men have difficulty in recognizing the female orgasm, how a man can discover a woman's sexual fantasies, and how men are altering their attitudes to women.

Boys of fifteen have bought the idea that they are supposed to know everything about sex. So when a boy is sixteen and his father takes him aside and says, "Son, there are some things you ought to know about screwing," the kid will pull a big bluff and tell his dad that he knows it all. Then he fumbles his way through his first two or three sexual encounters—and if they are good for him, he will stick to that way of sex for the rest of his life. He may only be fifty percent right in what he is doing, but the woman will go along with it, because she too has bought her own brand of folklore—that the man is expected to know everything about sex. So you get couples marrying early, living together for thirty years, doing the same thing in sex— and being unhappy about it.

How should a man learn to have sex?

A boy should start early and learn sexual technique in high school—with high-school girls who are also practicing. A boy can read sex manuals, but he should realize that they only teach the mechanics, which are like the finger exercises one learns when starting to play the piano. You do the finger exercises when you are fourteen or fifteen. The finger exercises are the mechanics, but the mechanics don't become music until you are so familiar with those mechanics that you express your feelings as well. By the time a boy is an adult he should have mastered technique and be into expressing feelings. The trouble is that too many men never get past the technique stage—they never forget the sex manual, "First you fondle the left breast, then you fondle her right breast, then you play with her clitoris and vagina—and when it's wet you put your penis in." Then they follow that program for the rest of their lives. An old routine.

What problems do those old routines cause?

I see many men who are disturbed because the girls they date now are no longer playing games or putting up with rituals and routines. I see the kind of man who is about fifty, high salary, sports car, nice apartment, wall-to-wall waterbed—the complete *Playboy* syndrome. He has always been used to taking a girl out to an expensive dinner, taking her home to his apartment, mixing the martinis, then putting the right romantic music on the stereo. Next smooching her neck, fondling her left breast, her right breast—going through the sex manuals. But nowadays the girl will say something like "This is kind of schoolgirl—let's have a nice friendly fuck," or "Look—it's ten-thirty and I've got to go to work tomorrow. Let's go to bed now." Then the man—who up till that moment has had a hard-on—becomes as limp as a rag. The girl has ruined his routine—he hasn't fondled her breasts, hasn't felt her vagina, doesn't know whether she is wet or dry—and the man can't function without his routine. Men like that need to retain the initiative sexually. Otherwise they become impotent, because they believe the *man* is supposed to decide when to have sex.

Does the routine-ridden man worry about the woman's orgasms?

Yes. Many of the men I see come to me because their world has fallen apart. They have suddenly encountered a woman who didn't orgasm but who said things like: "I don't want you to be offended—but when I get this turned on I frequently have to help myself to orgasm," or "I have a little trouble—would you mind if I masturbated?" Whereupon the man becomes impotent. I never tell men like that that their previous partners have probably been faking. It *is* difficult for a man to recognize a woman's orgasms—women with well-developed muscles can fake easily. In fact, women have said things like: "I got one of those bedroom athletes who wanted to go on for two hours—I get bored after forty-five minutes—so not only did I fake the orgasm, but I also squeezed the man so hard with my vaginal muscles that he came too." When I see men who are shattered because their last few partners haven't faked, I just say, "So, you met three nonorgasmic women in a row—the law of averages finally caught up with you." *Not* that most of their women have probably faked. The problem is that men like that aren't really into sex for sex's sake. They've been measuring their manhood by the efficiency of someone else's nervous system. Sex was an ego trip—in which they split off a piece of their personality, put it on the mantelpiece, and watched themselves. "Hey, Bruce, you've really done a good job, that's her fifth orgasm." They weren't relating to the woman—they were manipulating another body for responses which satisfied their own ego and made them feel like good sexual technicians. They were more interested in laying a woman than in laying *that particular* woman, and a woman feels it when a man is that way—she feels he is treating her like a thing, like the thing he was in bed with the night before.

What advice would you give to men like that?

He should pay attention to a woman's responses—consider her feelings. As early as possible. After he is in bed with her, he should say something like: "This is very important to me; I like you a lot and I want to be invited back. If I am doing something you like, or if I'm not doing something you like, or if I'm doing something you don't like, please tell me."

How should a man tell a woman if he wants something special?

If a man happens to have a fetish—like, say, bondage—he should wait until after about the first dozen fucks, then say: "I've got this quirk . . ." But if he can't function at all without bondage, he should break it to the woman before they go to bed the first time. It's unfair to go to bed with a woman without being honest. A man should always be willing to risk a piece of ass with honesty. Sexual communication is still awful today, in bed and out.

What is the cause of that?

Again, sexual routines, men going through the bullshit they've been developing since they were twelve. Some guys learn out of novels, others out of *True Confessions*, others out of *Playboy*. Then at school they discover a certain approach yields them a better return—so they stick to it. People always do stick with the last successful solution, which is why women have to cope with guys who come on with the same bullshit they read in *Playboy* fifteen years ago. Or you get a guy who, when he was growing up, found that he scored most by appealing to a woman's maternal instinct. As the years went by he never changed his lines or updated his techniques—so you end up with a fifty-five-year-old potbellied guy still going around trying to appeal to a woman's maternal instincts. Men like that are not lust-oriented, or relationship-oriented, but fuck-oriented. They were brought up to believe they gained status by fucking—whereas girls are educated to believe they lose status by fucking. So their objective is always scoring, pussy, and never getting to know a woman. Because they want to get screwed they feel they need to go around being nice to women. Then if they find one being nice back to them, they produce their full range of techniques in order to get into her pants. The majority of men in the U.S. don't really like women and feel that women are a race of wide-bottomed creatures they have to get along with in order to get laid. I would say that that is true of the average American over twenty-six, but there is an improvement in young people—and I am at last meeting young people of both sexes who are much more ready to see each other as human beings.

Pauline Abrams:
On More Male Sexual Problems

Pauline Abrams works as a sex therapist in New York; she treats both men and women. I asked her to discuss the physical and emotional problems from which her male patients suffer. Her interview is both factual and personal, dealing with the major mistakes made by men, male sexuality related to age, men and endowment, men and oral sex, and why men are beginning to feel more responsible for female pleasure. I began by asking Pauline Abrams to isolate the specific male problems caused by today's sexual climate.

Far too many men go to bed because there is a woman around who says yes. It's time men learned that you don't go to bed with a woman just because she's available. Sex for men today is like being in a candy store when they can eat as much as they want—it's easy for men to go to bed with women nowadays. So men either use a lot of willpower, or they go through the process of eating too much candy and discovering that gorging themselves indiscriminately just makes them sick. They end up in bed with

women they don't like—don't get erections and then
wonder why they're impotent!

What type of sexual problems do men face today?

The media have introduced men to the idea that
women are sexual beings who require sexual satisfaction just as men do. As a result men have become
aware that it's not enough to have intercourse, that
when a man goes to bed he has a responsibility to give
his woman pleasure. When I was a young girl I used to
fantasize that I was in a wealthy sultan's harem, being
trained to make superb love. The idea of being taught
to make love so that I would know what I was really
doing excited me. I think that men today are beginning
to have that same fantasy and want to learn how to
turn women on. Many patients I see are aware that
they are ignorant about female physiology and don't
know how to be good lovers—and that realization is
making a lot of men very nervous and dysfunctional.

*What are the specific problems for which you treat
your patients?*

I see men who are worrying about being good in
bed—but they don't express it that way; they say
things like "I am having difficulty getting erections" or
"I don't really know what turns a woman on." One
category we treat frequently is the premature ejaculator. These men enjoy sex and would like to last longer
for the woman. Unfortunately it is always for the
woman—never for themselves. If they wanted to last
longer for themselves they probably wouldn't be prematurely ejaculating at all, because their own sexuality
would motivate and drive them. Some premature ejaculators want the orgasm of the moment—rather than
putting it off till later for greater pleasure. They are often selfish and ejaculate because it feels good to them.
We teach them the ability to recognize the moment of
ejaculatory inevitability. There is a period of time be-

fore the man is about to come when he has enough time to stop himself, and he needs to be aware of that moment. Once the man recognizes the moment of ejaculatory inevitability, it is very easy for him to stop himself ejaculating by not continuing whatever he is doing.

What other sexual problems do men encounter?

Men worry a lot about penis size. I know that in my own personal sexual growth I've changed my mind about penis size several times. I used to say size didn't matter as I didn't want men who were small to feel bad. Then I met a few men who were great lovers *and* more than adequately endowed. So I got used to the vaginal experience of having sex with men who had above-average-size penises. It felt great so I decided that the size of a man's penis was just as important to a woman as the size of a woman's breasts to a man. Then I met a man with an average-size penis. He totally controlled the fucking, pushing me, pulling me, moving my legs and my body—totally controlling. He definitely wasn't a sensual man—the most important thing was intercourse—and I loved it. I discovered as well that I had a very sensitive cervix and that one of the advantages of being with a man with an average to small penis is that there were all sorts of positions that would give me pleasure—like doggy style or my legs over the man's shoulders. I can't do any of these if the man has a large penis, because then those positions would be painful.

Does the man with a large penis have more sexual self-confidence or does he try less? In What Makes A Woman G.I.B.? *many men said that a beautiful woman is less good in bed because she feels she doesn't have to do much because of her beauty—is there a parallel between a beautiful woman and a man with a large penis?*

No, I don't think so. Men with large penises generally seem to have better-developed egos and this does make them fuck better because they don't have concerns about size. As a result they are rarely dysfunctional, nor do they have any virility or premature ejaculation problems. However, they do sometimes worry that young girls won't go to bed with them because they are too well endowed. Also a man with a large penis knows that he has to compensate for those positions he's too big for by being very sensuous. In contrast, a man with a small penis must learn to give the woman sensations with his attack and delivery.

Male prostitutes for women stress the importance of giving oral sex to a woman—do you agree?

It is totally impossible for a man to be good in bed if he doesn't give a woman oral sex. Men who don't go down on women generally fear or experience that women don't smell good. Or they imagine that giving head won't give *them* any enjoyment. Kissing is pleasurable for a man because he gets kissed back— but some men can't see why sticking their tongues in a woman's vagina will give them pleasure. And too many men don't have the technical ability to give good oral sex.

How would you define good oral sex?

If a man is good at giving oral sex he turns a woman on to such an extent that her being turned on turns him on and the experience becomes mutual. The man has to do it with a passion—because he feels that giving a woman oral sex is as important as having intercourse with her, not just because he feels that the woman *wants* him to give oral sex. One of the biggest failings in men who give head is that they either lick the clitoris and don't lick the vagina or vice versa. The vagina is much more complicated than the male genitals, and all of it is arousable—not just the clitoris.

Is the quality of a man's sexuality recognizable when you first meet him?

I don't think so—and that is the big tragedy. Try as I might I have never been able to determine much about someone's sexuality before bed. Personalities are not indicative of sexual essences. I have met men who were marvelous lovers, but out of bed were highly neurotic individuals with whom one wouldn't want to spend much time. Then there were other men who were everything I wanted out of bed, but once in bed were nothing. The only indication is that sometimes there is a feeling of sexual energy that emanates from someone.

How does age determine a man's sexuality?

Being young and virile is not enough. A man also needs to have a certain experience. Eighteen-to-thirty-year-old men have marvelous virility but often lack control. But if the woman is very skilled she will reach a man at the height of his passion, physically at his best. Between thirty and forty the man is experienced but he can often be negatively affected by his experiences. Bad experiences can cause a man to become dysfunctional. If a man has never experienced a really fantastic female lover, he has less chance of being a good lover himself. So that by the time the man is in his forties his sexual development will have been determined. When a man is in his fifties he will take longer to have erections, he will be less cerebrally turned on and will need more tactile stimulation. Men in their fifties last longer, don't ejaculate so fast or so frequently, and the power of the ejaculate is lessened. However, a man in his fifties should have developed more skill and should know how to handle a woman psychologically—which will make him a better lover.

What do you personally think makes a man G.I.B.?

Ideally one wants a man who is tremendously sensual and has total abandonment when fucking. The man should be very loving, very sensual, not genitally oriented but very concerned with touch and sensitivity, knowing that the tongue and the mouth and the hands are as important as the penis. There are some men who are not like that at all. They get erections with ease, can maintain them for hours, and are perfectionists at intercourse only. Such a man becomes a perfectionist if he fucks a lot, if intercourse is his only motivation and goal of pleasure. I have had men who were totally useless in bed—except in intercourse; then they were great. Men like that are obsessed by fucking, not touching; they ride you, are driven by the need to fuck you. I don't think their attack and delivery is learnable—it is the result of tremendous sexuality and passion.

My final advice to both men and women who want to be good in bed is to be obsessed by sex. Great lovers are obsessed by sex and continually try to improve their sex lives. There is no question of being half-hearted. People who are great in bed are obsessed by sex—just as Picasso was obsessed by art. But sex has to be more important to you than art, than the movies, than the theater, and if it is, I am sure you will not only be good at it but will be great in bed.

What is your advice to the man who wants to be G.I.B.?

If a man wants to be G.I.B. he should learn about female anatomy. He should always remember that women are most turned on by being sexually related to as unique individuals. Women are most turned on when they feel that a man is relating to them in a specific way—a way in which he would never relate to anyone else. A man can impress on a woman how uniquely he is relating to her by the way in which he touches her face and vagina. If a man touches a woman's face with a tremendous amount of love, and care, and passion, and tenderness, the woman will feel personally related to. She will feel that way even more if the man looks at her vagina as if he enjoys looking at it as much as he does her face. As if her vagina were a thing of beauty—not something that just gave sexual pleasure, as if he was *obsessed* with her vagina. Any man who creates that feeling in a woman has definitely got her.

Dr. James Hemming: On Male Sexual Trends

Dr. James Hemming is a British social psychologist who is a noted observer of sexual trends. I asked him about specific problems men face when approaching women, the relationship between sex and age, and his general advice to men. The interview begins with Dr. Hemming's comments on media standards of sexuality.

We are no longer sure by which rules people are playing the sex game. We are now more free, but we often don't know what to do as individuals. The old taboos have gone, but I think we need to formulate some new rules by which to play the mating game in the modern world.

"Good in bed" is an artificial standard which has emerged from the spate of sexual material of all kinds that has poured over us in recent years. The media projects standards of sexuality. Both men and women measure themselves against an assumed absolute standard derived from the plays and films they see, the books they read, and then feel doubtful about whether they are meeting this standard.

The whole idea of "good in bed" and "super sex"—the idea that sex ought to be superlative at all times—has created an expectation of perfection which no one has fully defined. So everyone is chasing a fantasy, and the expectation of perfect sexual performance leads to each partner being nervous about whether they are good or not. I think that the glamorization and commercialization of sex is doing a lot of damage to sexual happiness as many men and women are now terribly afraid that they may be falling short in their sexual performance.

Sex today is often difficult for men because they are facing the increased confidence and effectiveness of women. It used to be easy for men to feel virile, sexually potent, the great ones, because women depended on them for a meal ticket. So men used to be born with a bonus of significance *because* they were male. Nowadays, men are losing ground in terms of power and significance because women are gaining it. There is a relationship between potency and confidence, so that if you take away the easy access to confidence and power, you are likely to detract from the sexual assurance of men. Many men feel insecure as a result of no longer being able to cash in on their former certainty of superiority.

Many modern girls won't fall for the old masculine line anymore. That line was "I'm male, I'm strong, I'm tough, I'm dominant." In the past, apart from being there, and from being masculine, men never needed to bother much. But today's relationships between men and women are becoming compassionate, rather than dominant/submissive. And if a man and a woman are involved in a compassionate relationship on equal terms, then each partner has to be concerned about what the other is feeling.

How do you define the problems men face when approaching women?

Men are still brought up believing that there is a series of magical things they can do to a woman that will lead her into submission and orgasm. Society has always suggested to men that women should be very accommodating so men get very upset if they are rejected. The common idea is, I am alone with a woman so I *ought* to make love to her. But the man who makes as many propositions as there are opportunities to make them is bound to be rejected on many occasions—and runs the risk of getting put down and dejected. Sexuality should be selective. Even animals are sexually selective. If a man propositions too many women, he will eventually get badly hurt. Some men become clumsy or impotent as a result of rejection. Men also often suffer from a lack of subtlety and need to realize that you can't play a violin with a sledgehammer. Some women like to be wooed, and an oversensitive man may interpret the woman's desire to be wooed as rejection.

Are male sexual problems age related, in terms of psychology?

The young male lacks understanding—he often feels he is doing all the right things, yet the sex doesn't seem to be working out. He is then forced into uncertainty: "*Have* I got it right now? Is there something I haven't learned?" He begins to wonder whether there is something other men are doing sexually that he is not. But by the time a man is in his late twenties he will probably be more confident. Also today's young male is beginning to realize that he can't be insensitive, that he has to learn about this strange feeling world that women inhabit, which up till now he has been taught *not* to inhabit. The older man is unlikely to be as frequent a lover or as enduring a lover in physical terms.

His erections won't come so readily or last as long. He won't always be in the mood for sex—but he will always be in the mood for a relationship. The older man is more appreciative of what "female" and "feminine" mean. Physically the older man will operate at a quieter tempo, but he will make up for what he lacks in virility by subtlety, warmth, gentleness, and appreciation. If a woman wants a lot of physical sex, stamina, and long periods of erection, she should remember that she is more likely to get these with a younger man than with an older one.

What advice would you give to the man who wants to be good in bed in a woman's judgment?

I prefer the phrase "A person who is good to be in bed with." If men are fairly secure, not rushing the sex, and not trying to prove their potency, then they will not find sex too difficult. But the man who thinks sex is routine behavior is too crude to be a successful lover. A man has got to be aware of the woman, of her moods and her needs. Men should treat each going to bed as a unique occasion.

A man should be tender, sensitive, and exploratory. Quite often the man still has to tempt the woman into new possibilities. Some women still feel guilty about uninhibited sexuality, so if the woman is nervous about any experimentation, the man shouldn't rush her, but instead should gradually expand her range of response so that he finally leads her toward new modes of experience.

I believe that it is very important for the man and the woman to communicate. There should be gentle communication in bed by gesture or touch, and the expressing of pleasure when you feel it. Little verbal promptings help, like "That's lovely" or "Not so hard." However, bed is an emotional and not a linguistic area, so that I think that sexual problems and desires should be discussed *before* bed. In an area as sensitive as sex

you should pave the way in general terms, asking
what sort of sexual experience the other person likes in
bed. Then the partner will usually respond by asking in
return.

Unfortunately people are often bashful about discussing what they like in bed, believing it will show they
are "no good." Of course you can go to bed and
chance it. But it seems very curious to me that a man
and a woman often go to bed with each other without
knowing anything about each other's expectations. Sex
is the only situation in which we act like this. If two
people plan to go on a holiday together, they discuss
what they like first—"Do you like the mountains? Do
you like the sea?"—and I think they should do the
same when they go to bed.

Each partner should tell the other in good time anything they dislike sexually, but at the same time should
add, "What I really do like is *this*." So that one builds,
giving something back if one has taken something
away. I personally believe that "good in bed" is a part-
nership, not a person. It's not what you do, it's how
you relate. And that is very much a here and now
thing of being sensitive to the person you are in bed
with. Every sexual experience is really an exploration
of the other partner and should be highly reciprocal.
People wear masks, and behind each mask is a much
frailer, much more needful, much more insecure person. And the partner who is "good" takes off their
mask and as it were, says, "Here I am—a needful human being ready to love you."

Kate Lloyd:
On How Men Are Coping with the
Liberated Woman

Kate Lloyd epitomizes the liberated woman. A graduate of Bryn Mawr, winner of the Prix de Paris, a former managing editor of *Vogue*, the mother of two children, she looks like the French actress Jeanne Moreau and is managing editor of the magazine *Working Woman*. Kate Lloyd deals daily with letters from working women all over America, and I interviewed her on how men are coping with the new liberated woman, whether or not that woman rates men sexually, what her effect on men is, and what the liberated woman really wants from a man in bed.

I think there is a new generation of women now in their twenties who did not grow up with the same hangups and rules of the game that I did. I grew up in what was really an echo of the Edwardian culture—although it was in the 1940s. I don't think my mother told me anything about sex. I learned through school chums, so that by the time my mother got around to telling me, it was too late. I was already loaded with misinformation, and clichés were hanging off me like Christmas-tree ornaments. At that time it wasn't nice to have an affair—men wouldn't respect you if you went to bed with them. Flirting was the only way of communication between men and women—and in a way flirting was fun.

Nowadays there is an enormous directness—everything is so simple—almost no mating dance, no courtship or flirtation. The game has gone. Young people today have grown up without experiencing any taboos. For example, boys and girls live together in co-educational fraternities and dormitories and lose their hang-ups as a result. They watch each other grow up and become aware of each other's frailties. This puts men and women into a position of equality as human beings, which also reflects itself sexually. I think women have lost the discomfort my generation felt when they were with men. That discomfort came from knowing—if only subconsciously—that a woman's economic survival depended on her relationship with a man.

Now that many women don't need to depend on men for economic survival, they are free from having to listen to everything that they do in terms of "Am I doing this right in order to catch a fellow?"

Does a new woman exist who is rating men sexually?

Yes—but not in a clinical way. I doubt if many women are really comparing notes on men. But I do think that women who used to feel it was criminal even to think about how men are in bed are beginning to think, "Gee—that was great," or, "Gee—that wasn't great." I still find it hard though to imagine sex on a clinical "I need sex" level. And from what I see of my own kids and their friends, they do too. I think it is the age group between mine and my children's—the thirties—who are involved in swinging.

What effect do you think the change in women is having on men?

I think the younger men who grew up in this new climate are comfortable with it, and with the new approach of women. But I think that older men sometimes feel very threatened and slightly confused. Men who are older are still used to dealing with women on the level of "she gives/he takes"—so that they often get distressed by the abruptness and nonchalance of the young women of today.

How would you advise older men to cope with the new woman?

An older man should treat a woman as if she were a human being. We should tell men the truth: "You are no smarter than a woman is—you don't need to be approached in an old-fashioned, coquettish way—you ought to be able to accept the fact that you are being communicated with as a human being, not with any window dressing." One could still tell men, "For a person of your experience, your intelligence, your worldly wisdom—just help these women a little by putting up with the passing fancies they are going through. You have the clout—the machismo—to help them over it." That kind of an approach may make relationships between some insecure men and women easier, but it will be a dishonest approach, and therefore a dishonest relationship.

Fifteen years ago when a woman refused a man, he could tell himself, "Fine, she is a virgin—she doesn't." Today there is very little a man can tell himself if the woman refuses. How is that affecting men when they are rejected?

I think men felt equally rejected by women even when they had the panacea of "Oh well—she is a virgin." The feeling of the chase hasn't changed at all, and men still feel equally rejected. I don't think that human beings ever think of themselves as anything other than the exception—so that it didn't matter if the woman's excuse was that she was a virgin, because every man felt that he should be the exception and that the woman should lose her virginity to him. So that the sense of rejection for men was equally great then as now.

If you could create the composite man for the new liberated woman—what do you think she wants?

I think that the liberated woman's ideal still contains a lot of romantic elements. We always did want a man to be handsome and strong and intelligent and protective. I don't think that has changed terribly much—except that we now want a lot of other things as well. We want emotional and physical support—in the sense of the man helping to take on some of the chores if both partners work. I think we also expect tenderness from the man. The "Me Tarzan—you Jane" routine is ridiculous and phony. The exchange of tender feelings is very important to the liberated woman. She is now out on a kind of firing line and needs a loving and understanding person to come home to—just as men always have done.

What advice would you give to men on how to be good in bed for the new liberated woman?

I would tell them to relax and enjoy it. I think there is sometimes too much arming. You don't arm yourself for sex. And if you feel you have to—forget it.

Dr. Herb Goldberg: On Sex and the Liberated Man

Dr. Herb Goldberg is a Los Angeles psychologist and author of *The Hazards of Being Male*, which examines the phenomenon of the liberated male. I asked him to define different categories of men: the macho man, the sadistic man, the masochistic man, the powerful man—and, of course, the liberated man. He also discussed the ways in which woman's liberation is affecting sexuality, situations which create sexual pressure for men, and causes of male sexual insecurity.

First of all I hate the phrase "good in bed" because it implies servicing. But I think some people use the phrase about themselves. A man more than anything else rates *himself*—whether *he* thinks he is good in bed. A macho man rates a sexual experience by the woman's response—how many orgasms she has had, how long he has controlled his orgasm, how long he has maintained his erection. He is actually proving things to himself. When a macho male says a sexual experience was good, I say, "What did *you* get out of it?" and he looks befuddled and cannot answer.

Is the new liberated woman affecting male sexuality?

There is less pressure for men to perform nowadays because many women are no longer playing the old passive, submissive roles. They are beginning to take responsibility for their own orgasm and are more into men as people rather than as performers. But in another way there is more pressure. I see men all the time who have these problems within the framework of a committed relationship. Suddenly a wife or girlfriend becomes infused with feminine consciousness—goes through a reawakening, a liberation, and realizes that she has never had an orgasm or that her orgasms have not been deep enough or often enough. So for the first time in her life she asserts herself and makes conscious demands: "Hey, I haven't been getting enough out of this—I want you to start satisfying me." This puts pressure on the man. If the crisis occurs after many years of marriage, the man frequently can't handle it and withdraws.

Does this situation cause impotence?

I don't use the words "impotence" or "dysfunction" because they both imply performance standards. Whenever a guy tells me, "I am impotent," I say to him, "Please substitute for the word 'impotence' the phrase 'I don't want to make love to that particular woman.'" Primary impotence, which means never getting an erection with any woman, is very rare. Most so-called impotence is selective impotence. The man can make it very well with one woman but not with another. That is not impotence but a body statement.

What other kind of situations create sexual pressure for the man?

If the man feels he is in competition with other men for a particular woman and that she is a trophy that other men want, he will be under sexual pressure. Or if he finds the woman that he has always been looking for—and wants to prove his masculinity. That is when even the most liberated man finds the woman he thinks is the magic lady of his dreams, he tends to regress to pounding his chest and proving what a man he is. Then there is a situation where a man who has been monogamous for a long time gets divorced and is unsure of himself and has to reassure himself sexually. Or an older man with a younger woman feels he has to perform in bed to keep up with the younger guys. All these circumstances can be loaded with performance anxieties for the man. Especially if he is a macho male.

How do you define the macho male?

The macho male makes love to an object—not a woman. He has too much performance anxiety to feel his own feelings—too much anxiety to allow the woman's feelings to really emerge. Frequently he needs to be dominant. He will ask the woman if she has had an orgasm. He will look for reassurance about his performance. He will be very sensitive about any negative criticism or discussion about his sexuality. He will probably be very careful with his language if he thinks he is in love. He is extremely vulnerable to the madonna/whore complex in dividing women up into two groups—the woman he loves and the woman he screws. He feels a great pressure to live up to the masculine role image—to suppress emotion, weakness and vulnerability, not to allow himself to be dependent or submissive. To always have an erection, to please a woman, to be in control and be dominant.

How can a man be dominant and please a woman? Surely dominant implies the man doing what he wants and not what the woman wants?

It is very easy, because in his fantasies the man thinks that the woman wants him to be dominant. Men like that end up thinking they are great lovers. Those are the men for whom women fake. When women talk about macho men they say things like "I want to tell him how I really feel, but I don't want to threaten him, so I will pretend to have an orgasm." So they fake because they know that the macho man is defensive and insecure in his sexuality.

Can you pinpoint the cause of other male sexual insecurities?

The trouble is that some men make too great a distinction between behavior out of bed and behavior in bed. I think they are one and the same thing. A lot of men who have nothing in common with a woman out of bed expect to have a highly sexual experience with her in bed. A man who will not talk to a woman very much out of bed, who is not playful with her in the living room, expects suddenly to get into bed with her and become playful. Or a man who doesn't enjoy touching, smelling, looking at, and listening to his girlfriend as they walk through the streets expects a whole new consciousness to prevail once they are between the sheets. But sex is nothing more than an extension of the interaction outside of bed.

How does that apply to men who go to prostitutes and are satisfied sexually by them?

Going to a prostitute is the ultimate form of male self-hate and humiliation. On an unconscious level going to a prostitute is a masochistic experience, paying her to make love to you.

Can you give me a profile of a masochistic man?

Masochistic men are attracted to women who are basically rejecting. A rejecting woman fits into his masculine conditioning because she creates a constant challenge—and challenge is what men are brought up to be excited by. Many men will go from woman to woman until they find a woman who dominates them emotionally—who they need a lot more than she needs them. They want a woman who controls the situation, creating a perpetual sense of excitement and challenge. So that the man never knows for sure where he stands, or if she will go off with another man the next day. This creates a permanent sexual high.

Can you profile the sadistic man?

Sadism may take many different forms—"detachment," refusal to engage and participate actively, treating a woman like an object. A sadistic man is indifferent to a woman, insensitive to her needs. A great deal of masculine behavior can look like sadism; men have been taught to repress and deny their aggression toward women—particularly if they're in love. Then they treat women like queens—like fragile flowers. Consequently, in a typically romantic relationship, the male represses a lot of his negative feelings. All of his aggression goes underground because he doesn't want to hurt the woman's feelings. But periodically the aggression emerges in indirect forms which can look like sadism: violent urges, sometimes involving actual physical abuse. This is because the man is dropped into a situation in which he is supposed to be the strong man, the protective man, the perfect lover, husband, and father. He plays that role because of his own sensibilities and thus accumulates a lot of anger and periodically explodes a buildup of resentment if the man is almost inequitable because of the constant pressure to perform he feels himself to be under.

What about men with power? What is the powerful man like in bed?

The powerful man in our society has to learn to manipulate and mask. Strong qualities of detachment and manipulation are not conducive to warm and intense relationships. Men who have power are very image-conscious. Consequently they operate on many levels—the public levels, and the private levels on which they are afraid to expose their real selves. So they are prone to having affairs in secret and degrading ways so that they can be real. They choose situations in which they are using the woman and the woman is using them.

What makes the liberated man good in bed?

I would rephrase that to: "What are the conditions that allow the liberated man to fulfill himself maximally in bed?" The best conditions for a man to fulfill himself in bed are those that allow him to be playful, free from any concern about his erection or the woman's orgasm, to be emotionally expressive, transparent with his fantasies, reactions, and responses, and very much in touch with his senses. He needs to be self-accepting, in touch with his emotions, in touch with himself, so that he easily expresses his needs, his feelings, and his fantasies. He needs to like himself so that he knows what he wants. To be aware of his senses and to choose women that bring out the playful in him, transcending role expectations and operating as a person rather than as a man. Operating from his needs and feelings. I think a woman will open up if the man opens up. If the man shares his fantasies, is comfortable with them, the woman will reveal her fantasies as well. Unless she is a very repressed or defensive woman. In that case I don't see it as the man's role to play therapist in bed. I don't see that reassuring each other is the role of either the male or the female in bed. The man shouldn't degrade the woman, or himself, by treating her like a fragile flower; he should assert his needs, and share his feelings. He should remember that both partners are free, responsible, and assertive people.

Letitia Baldrige ("Amy Vanderbilt"): On Male Sexual Etiquette

Letitia Baldrige has rewritten Amy Vanderbilt's book on etiquette, and I talked to her about sexual etiquette for men in the 1970s and 80s. Having encountered "California casual"—a European at sea in a country of singles bars, first-night seductions, and "I'll call you"—I wondered if any formality still existed in America and how this applied to men. Letitia Baldrige seemed the perfect person to ask. A graduate of Miss Porter's and Vassar, she was social secretary to the White House during President Kennedy's administration. I started the interview by asking her about the differences in etiquette in pre-Pill America.

In "other" days a lady would never talk about sex. There was no question of how we had to behave because there was a totally rigid moral structure. Women used to be moral, afraid of hurting their parents and afraid of getting pregnant. Therefore women were very strong about curbing their sexuality, fighting emotions and desires. Perhaps as a result, my generation finds it easier to cope with life in general, without feeling dispirited—because we have always been used to controlling our actions as related to our emotions. I sometimes wish I had the freedom of today's generation—but then again, I am glad I grew up when I did.

Is there a new sexual etiquette?

In the young, the rigid moral structure seems to have disappeared, but I don't think there are any new rules of sexual behavior. We are still in a state of flux because the women's movement has unsettled things, making women freer about what they want to do and when. Sex today comes about between two people who are fond of each other—without form, manners, or anything; with no pressure at all as to when, where, or how sex should happen.

Is a new sexual behavior emerging?

Yes. I think men and women are no longer afraid to say how they feel—when they are ready for sex and when they are not. The woman's movement of the 1960s was such a revolution—people are less hysterical, less pressured, in the '70s, and I think we have now reached a happy phase. I talk to many young people on campuses, and I think they are becoming more idealistic. They talk about love more—and plain old having fun. Girls used to tell me about being pressured to have sex—they felt they would be less popular if they refused. And boys sometimes told me that they felt the same. But I think all that is changing.

What is your advice to men regarding the etiquette of coping with the advances of a woman?

I think it is bad news for either a man or a woman to be predatory. It's thoughtless and inconsiderate for one person to try to rush the other into the bedroom. If a woman persists in that kind of an approach, a man should just simply rebuff her. It's a sign of gross insecurity if someone tries to pressure another person to go to bed. People who are secure and happy human beings, successful in their human relationships, don't apply pressure.

How do you think a man should approach a woman?

I don't think the first approach is a question of manners. It is a question of human response of one person to another, even a question of character. Some people are just not kind, considerate, or thoughtful about anyone else. And I firmly believe that sex should be a question of understanding how the other person feels and of being kind, and of responding to feelings and understanding nuances.

What kind of nuances should a man look for?

I'm talking about a man and his wife. It's a question of one person giving the cues and the other person responding. The way a hand is suddenly placed on another hand—little ways of showing love and responsiveness. Then the other person can say, "Yes—I think it is a great idea," or, "No—I have other things on my mind." I think it is sad when young girls and young men feel obliged to perform the minute they have the first date. Luckily, though, I think the woman's movement is changing all that.

What will you tell your children about sex?

I shudder to think what life is going to be like for my daughter. I won't expect her to behave as we did in my generation, because I know that today one can't demand that a girl remain a virgin unendingly. But I hope she will be a long time, and I hope she will never be promiscuous. I will tell my son to be kind and considerate—and beware of the double-standard. After all the woman still has the babies.

In a way, we are swinging back to yesterday, because a lot of young women are now afraid to take the Pill.

Above all, I will tell both my children that sex is part of love—because I don't think that good sex is possible without love.

What kind of sexual etiquette would you like to see emerging in the 1980s?

Peoples' behavior behind the bedroom door is *not* a question of etiquette! The major reason for having rules is happiness. And people should remember that everything they do stems from their character. If a person is a kind and thoughtful person, he or she is going to be a kind and thoughtful lover. And if a person is a selfish human being, he or she is going to be a selfish lover. People act the same way in their sexual lives as they do in their office lives, in their relationships with their children and other adults. Sexual manners are a matter of self-control, and of thinking about the other person. The result of good manners in *any* form of activity is usually happiness.

Dr. Erika Padan Freeman:
On Male Sexual and Emotional Differences

Dr. Erika Padan Freeman is one of the leading psychoanalysts in the Western world and the author of *Insights: Conversations with Theodore Reik*. She treats both men and women, so I asked her to define the differences between the sexes in terms of guilt, emotional involvement, relationship goals, approach, sincerity, and intuition. We also talked about sex related to profession, men with a madonna/whore complex, why men should never pounce on a woman, how men can read women, and man the hunter.

One of the major differences between men and women is that men are trained in the pleasure principle—and women are not. The result is that if a woman enjoys sex she feels guilty, and her guilt negates her enjoyment. Whereas most men are able to enjoy sex without guilt. But men do need sex with emotion—usually a man's most sensually and sexually superb experience will be with a woman he loves. Of course some men can also have very exciting sex with women they hate. But then hate is also an emotional involvement, and without emotional involvement you can't have superb sex. The depression men sometimes experience after sexual intercourse stems from having had sex without feeling.

There are some men who suffer from the madonna/whore complex; they are unable to have sex as part of a relationship with a woman they love. They feel that love and sex must be separate. Some women fantasize about also operating on a madonna/whore

basis in their relationships with men, but until we have
test-tube babies and women no longer are geared to
maternity, they will always need to feel related. A
woman never sleeps with a phallus—she always sleeps
with a man. Whereas many men sleep with vaginas, and
that is why they are able to say, "They are all the same
in the dark," but there isn't a woman in the world who
can say the same about men and mean it.

No matter what a woman says, she is always looking
for a relationship of some duration. Whereas a man is
looking for a conquest, and in order to conquer he will
say whatever is necessary. The clever seducer will always say what the woman wants to hear; that he loves
her, that he will stay with her, cherish her, and always
care about her. Men are forever implying everything
that women forever are listening for. One of the biggest
mistakes women make is to take a man at his word.
Whereas the biggest mistake a man makes is not to
take a woman at her word. Women usually say what
they mean—if a woman says she isn't interested in a
man, there is a strong possibility that she isn't.

Women are more intuitive than men—more able to
read body language and interpret unspoken sexual pre-
liminaries. So that it is important for a man to reflect
what he really feels. Women like finesse. They have a
sense of continuity and want a relationship to have a
beginning, a middle, and an end. Men should never
pounce suddenly, because a woman relates pouncing to
rape. The pouncing approach would work only if the
woman has indicated that she wants to go to bed immediately. It is very important for a man to discover a
woman's sexual desires. The men who know how to
read women are able to do so because they really care.
They don't treat a woman like an object, because they
know that if a woman is treated like a chair she won't
ever communicate—you don't expect a chair to communicate. And communication is not exclusively limited to words. Sexual vocabulary is also eye contact,
body language, physical contact, and ambience.

Artists, writers, and most creative men are usually better in bed, because they are more intuitive and gentle, and thus more sensitive to a woman's reactions and say, "If I do this, that will happen." Actors are also good in bed, unless they are too narcissistic and want to be deified. They have a feminine component and so understand how to please a woman. But if a man is too obsessed by his goal-oriented profession he is often subject to strain which will affect his sexuality. And if a man is obsessed with an occupation it becomes eroticized—his sexuality is no longer directly sexual because all his sexual energy is channeled into his obsession, so that the obsession becomes his real mistress.

The only way to have a good sexual relationship is to give oneself entirely. I don't think men know how to give of themselves. But some men do try in various ways. If a man who defines his worth by money gives a woman money, then he is giving of himself by giving something that he thinks is valuable. And if a man who defines himself by his work tells a woman about it, he too is giving of himself. A man can also give by letting the woman know how much he desires her. Desire is the turn-on which makes the woman feel worthwhile. Unfortunately a woman judges herself by a man's opinion of her—she will think he is good in bed if he tells her *she* is.

Men need to redefine their attitudes in order to be good in bed. They have to learn to depend on women—because up till now men have been taught to depend only on each other, in the army, on the sports field etc. Men still retain the value system of the ancient hunter: go out, hunt, bring it back, and rest. That value system has nothing to do with human relationships. But I think that the old hunter's values must soon disappear, because there aren't many places left to go hunting, to be all that physical about. And perhaps men may once again adopt the Greek ideals of leisure, of excellence of the mind, of knowledge, and of human relationships. Then men will learn that they don't have to say, "Of course I love you—I have hunted and here is the carcass"—that they don't *have* to bring back a carcass every time—because they themselves are what really matters to a woman.

Dr. Erika Padan Freeman's interview ends on a hopeful note for the future. There are conclusions about male sexuality in the present that can be drawn from the experts, and I have listed the points made under the following headings: Summary of Male Sexual Problems, Summary of Male Sexual Mistakes, Summary of Sexual Advice to Men, Summary of What Women Want Sexually.

SUMMARY OF MALE SEXUAL PROBLEMS

1. Inability to express feelings and desires.
2. Inadequacy in interpreting female sexuality.
3. Difficulty in concentrating on a woman.
4. Inability to have sex within the context of a relationship.
5. Fear of sexual failure.
6. Fear of not living up to mythical sexual standards.
7. Ignorance of the facts of sex.
8. Worrying about penis size.
9. Feeling nervous about one's own sexual performance.
10. Inability to feel virile if the woman is economically independent.
11. Feeling defensive and sexually insecure.
12. Feeling pressured to perform sexually.
13. Feeling distressed because of female openness.
14. Disturbed by woman demanding orgasms.
15. Fear of rejection.
16. Being pressured into having sex by the woman.
17. Fear of being compared unfavorably sexually.

18. Low sex drive.
19. Feeling guilt and anxiety because of upbringing.
20. Difficulty in coping with a woman who wants to bring herself to orgasm.
21. Difficulty in recognizing a female orgasm.
22. Inability to give oral sex.
23. Premature ejaculation.
24. Being negatively affected by bad sexual experiences.
25. Inability to have good sex with a loved woman.
26. Obsession with an occupation, so that all sexual energy is channeled into the occupation.
27. Inability to give of oneself.
28. Distrusting women out of fear of being possessed.

SUMMARY OF
MALE SEXUAL MISTAKES

1. Being too sexually goal-oriented.
2. Pressuring a woman into bed.
3. Approaching a woman insensitively.
4. Going to bed indiscriminately and failing.
5. Sticking to techniques and forgetting emotion.
6. Sticking to sexual routines.
7. Always needing to take the initiative sexually.
8. Insisting that the woman always orgasm.
9. Trying to score the woman instead of getting to know her.
10. Not giving a woman oral sex.
11. Lack of subtlety.
12. Using sex as a means of proving masculinity.
13. Asking the woman if she has had an orgasm.
14. Going to bed with women they don't like.
15. Always wanting to have simultaneous orgasms.
16. Setting too high a sexual standard for oneself.
17. Pretending to know a lot about sex and not trying to learn.
18. Making sex into an ego trip.

19. Wanting to have sex in general, not with a particular woman.
20. Sticking to lines learned from a sex magazine.
21. Never updating sexual techniques.
22. Viewing sex as a means of gaining status.
23. Pouncing on a woman.
24. Concentrating on the sex and forgetting about the relationship.
25. Rating oneself by the number of times the woman orgasms.
26. Suppressing emotion.
27. Propositioning too many women and becoming impotent as a result of rejection.

SUMMARY OF
SEXUAL ADVICES TO MEN

1. Don't hurry.
2. Concentrate on your feelings and the woman's.
3. Communicate through body and words.
4. Approach a woman nonverbally with a sexual gesture that is nonsexual, like touching the woman's hand.
5. Don't go to bed with a woman unless you are sure she wants to.
6. Try to recognize the type of woman you are in bed with.
7. Don't try to prove your potency.
8. Treat each going to bed as a unique occasion.
9. Be tender, sensitive, and exploratory.
10. Communicate gently.
11. Gradually lead the woman into new areas of experience.
12. Discuss sex before bed—not in bed.
13. Don't worry about the woman's orgasm or your erection.
14. Be emotionally expressive.
15. Be transparent with your fantasies.

16. Relax.
17. Watch the woman's reactions.
18. Communicate with eyes and body language.
19. Realize that not every woman is going to be right for you.
20. Try to communicate with a woman as an equal.
21. Talk fantasies to a woman—describe a series and ask which one she prefers.
22. Ask the woman to tell you what she likes or doesn't like.
23. If you can't function without a fetish, tell the woman before you go to bed with her the first time.
24. Learn about female anatomy.

SUMMARY OF
WHAT WOMEN WANT SEXUALLY

1. Tenderness.
2. A man who is concerned.
3. A man who is sensitive.
4. A man who has a feminine streak.
5. A man who is perceptive and aware.
6. A man they can talk to.
7. A man who is sexual.
8. A man who is assertive and strong.
9. To feel secure within a relationship.
10. To be loved one moment and raped the next.
11. A man who relates to them as unique individuals.
12. A good friend and an intimate companion.
13. Respect.
14. A man who is sensual and not genitally oriented.
15. A man who knows that the tongue and mouth and hands are as important as the penis.
16. Unbridled passion.
17. A man who gives oral sex because he wants to.
18. A man who is handsome, strong, intelligent and protective.

19. A man who gives emotional and physical support.
20. A relationship of some duration.
21. To hear that the man loves her, will stay with her and always care about her.

    The male interviewees that follow will confess to some of the problems and mistakes on the previous lists, sometimes echoing but other times disagreeing with the experts' advice. Later in the book the female interviewees reveal whether or not they agree with the experts' list of what women want. But first the generalizations of "the experts" are personalized by "the male celebrities."

Part II

The Male Celebrities

The anonymous men with problems and patterns discussed in the last section become personalized in this section, which presents "case histories" with a difference. That difference is that the case histories are some of America's most famous men—experiencing their sexual insecurities, their likes, dislikes, fantasies, their attitude to love, sex, and relationships, and their advice to other men.

Interviewee Selection

I have already explained my reasons for interviewing celebrities. I could provide data on my interviewees—their nationality, race, and creed. But their names and notoriety make all that unnecessary. The interviews are presented partly in age groups (but not in strict order of age) and also sometimes by nationality; for example, Giancarlo Giannini and Rossano Brazzi are together, to illustrate changes in attitude in Italian men.

Topics Discussed

Apart from advice to men, the major topics discussed by the male celebrities include sex in America today, "how I lost my virginity," how to approach a woman, how to find out what a woman wants sexually, the female orgasm, women's liberation, and the relationship between love and sex. The questions I asked will demonstrate other areas of discussion.

Questions to Interviewees

I asked the male celebrities questions I was curious about; questions on their image, their sexual preferences, problems and desires. These are the questions:

Hot Seat (103)

How did you lose your virginity?

How did you feel about that experience?

Did you lie about sex as a teenager?

Did you ever worry about being good in bed?

How do you think attitudes to sex in America have changed since you grew up?

What do you think your best sexual age was?

Do you think sexuality is inherent?

Do you ever feel pressured to be good in bed?

Do you ever not enjoy sex?

Do you like being told you are good in bed?

Do you think a man must always be ready to make love?

Has a woman ever made you feel sexually inadequate?

Do you like one-night stands?

What shocks you sexually?

How do you approach a woman?

How can you tell if she is attracted to you?

How do you feel if a woman approaches you?

Do you think a man should give a woman lots of compliments?

How would you advise a man to find out what a woman wants sexually?

How should a man communicate what he wants in bed?

Do you like a woman to initiate a new sex act?

Do you ever feel you have to live up to a sexy image?

Does your celebrity status give you self-confidence?

Do you think a woman should initiate sex?

Is it important for you if the woman has an orgasm?

Why is it important for you if the woman has an orgasm?

Do you mind if a woman fakes?

Can you tell if a woman fakes?

Do you feel bad if a woman fakes?

Do you still enjoy sex if the woman doesn't have an orgasm?

Do you think sex is important for a woman?

Do you think men and women get different degrees of pleasure out of sex?

Do you think women care if a man is a good lover?

What kind of a man do you think women want?

Do you think men masturbate more than women?

Do you need to feel a woman loves you before having sex with her?

Do you have to love a woman to have sex with her?

Is sex better with love?

How important do you think sex is to a relationship?

Has women's liberation changed your relationships with women?

Do you approve of women's liberation?

What do you think makes a man good in bed?

What advice would you give to other men who want to be good in bed?

What will you tell your children about sex?

Some of these questions have been left in the text of the interviews, to isolate the issue. I didn't ask every interviewee the same questions, but every one of the above questions is answered by the men in this section. Some of the questions are specific, others general; all are relevant questions designed for every woman to ask the man in her life. She can not only discover his attitudes, but also compare his answers to those of some of America's most famous men.

Richard Burton

In some ways I owe this book to Richard Burton. When I was fourteen years old I saw him filming *The Spy Who Came in from the Cold* in Battersea Park, London; he looked at me with searingly blue eyes, his voice rippled through me, and I fell in love with him.

Ten years later, now a journalist, I was sent by BBC radio to interview Burton. He was playing the part of Sir Winston Churchill in *A Walk with Destiny*, had just divorced Elizabeth Taylor for the first time, and I had already promised my friends diamonds. I was delivered into the presence of my idol, whose hair had been dyed white for the role of Churchill. Trembling, overflowing with emotion, adoration, and general gush, I stood clutching my little list of questions ("What was your favorite part?" "Why did you start acting?"), very much the junior journalist. Burton looked me up and down, and there was a moment's silence. Then he said, "I have a golden award for the first journalist who asks me a question I have never been asked before. And somehow, I don't think *you* are going to get it." Enthusiasm deflated, tremulous and tearful, I stumbled through my questions, consoled only by Richard Burton offering me half of a chocolate bar.

Later, I realized I had learned something from Richard Burton; celebrities are often bored by the same questions on their latest play, film, book, or record, and are prepared to discuss other subjects. The knowledge gave me the confidence to start my first book, *What Makes a Woman G.I.B.* I told Burton that when I eventually phoned him at his New York hotel, thanked him, and did this interview. I finally did ask Richard Burton a question he had never been asked before—but he still owes me his golden award.

Crown Prince of romance, womanizing Welshman, legendary lover, survivor of marriage, divorce, and scandal, Burton is very articulate and intellectual. As a published author, Richard asked me to make it clear that the interview was spoken, not written, and I suggest you "read it with the ear" and imagine Richard Burton's magnificent voice speaking the words. We talked mostly about his attitudes to sex and his approach to women. Burton was controlled, used precise language, corrected himself a lot, and was most gracious.

A quick, hasty "one-nighter" is too short a time to know the body of a woman. I was never the kind of chap who went to a party or a dance, picked up a girl, took her home, made love to her in the back of a car or in his apartment, then rolled over, went to sleep, or took the woman home. I've never understood that kind of man. The three wives and the few women—more than a few women, I'm afraid, when I was younger—all lasted a very long time.

I am actively repelled by the minds of girls who throw themselves around communes—have babies and no one knows the father. I wouldn't be at all interested in that type of girl. The woman who brings out the best in a man—who is good in bed—is very rare. In my entire life I have known only three. The qualities they possessed were a responding passion and a responding love.

The women's lib movement has definitely affected sexual attitudes—you can feel it in the air. There's a philosophy now that men are deliberately cultivating homosexuality as a defense against fem lib. Even the most feminine-looking woman is aware of the fem lib movement. Women like that are not going to be taken in by mellifluous voices saying set, cliché'd words.

You have to be very careful in approaching a woman in a cliché'd way—response varies according to the woman. Usually I think cliché'd words are probably best to use with any woman, unless she is excessively intelligent, or brusque or slightly lesbian. So the first thing you do with most women is to say how beautiful they are. Nine times out of ten it works. "Did anybody ever tell you you were a lovely girl?" "Did anybody ever tell you that your eyes were divine?" I think you can move ahead with clichés if you can smell, or physically see a counter-reflection in the eyes of the woman. You can recognize attraction in a woman's eyes because a woman's pupils dilate when she is attracted to a man—so that you can be fairly sure in advance whether you are going to be rebuffed or not.

I think some men are probably born to be more passionate than others. I know men, for instance, who are virgins at fifty—which I hardly am. Quite clearly, a cloistered life, like that of a don at Oxford—a pedantic life—might turn a man into a neuter. I know a great deal of those because I know Oxford very well. Also something might happen to make a man stray from the path, and even turn him into a homosexual. The passionate man obviously has a great start on the man who is merely amorous—and the hyperpassionate man has a great advantage over any of them because his sheer lust for the flesh is so much greater, and combined with love that becomes something extraordinary.

To succeed in the art of love a man must love the woman—that is the essence. You must first love, or *think* you love, the woman. When you are with *the only* woman—the only one you *think* there is for that moment—you must love her and know her body as if you were blind and your hands were reading braille. You must learn her body as you think a great musician would orchestrate a divine theme. You must use everything you possess—your hands, your fingers, your speech; seductively, poetically, sometimes brutally, but always with a demoniacal passion.

Sidney Sheldon

Sidney Sheldon, best-selling author of *The Other Side of Midnight*, *A Stranger in the Mirror*, and *Bloodline*, became a novelist after twenty-five years as a Hollywood screenwriter and producer. Aptly, I first met Sidney Sheldon in Hollywood, where we had lunch at the Bel Air Hotel. A year later we met again at the Regency Hotel in New York, where Sidney was having meetings about the Audrey Hepburn/Omar Sharif motion picture of *Bloodline*. While we talked a New York *Post* photographer snapped pictures of Sidney, who carried on discussing the subject, undaunted.

In his early sixties, married for over twenty years, Sidney Sheldon is debonaire, gentlemanly—the Cary Grant of best-selling authors. And if Richard Burton is a European romantic, then Sidney Sheldon is a regretful American, trying to discard traditional attitudes to woman and to sex, but nevertheless still reflecting them.

Men want to retain the illusion of women being fragile and delicate, vulnerable, and sometimes unattainable. Men aren't used to women who like sex—they are used to women being princesses. For centuries—from the beginning of time—the man has always been the aggressor—has hit the woman with his club and taken her back to his cave. A man got the food, hunted the animal, and was always the aggressor. So it takes time for men to get used to woman's new role of being as free and open about sex as men are.

If the woman's role has changed, what other changes in attitude to sex have you seen in recent years?

Twenty-five years ago I wrote a picture for MGM to which the censor refused a seal of approval. And without a seal of approval a picture could not be released. So I went to the censor's office to discuss the problem. The censor showed me the unacceptable scene. A man and a woman were in a room—the man pointed to two other characters also in the room, said, "I think they want to be alone," switched off the light, and left the room with the woman. The censor told me that before he would give the picture his seal of approval I would have to change that scene because it had sexual connotations. The two characters the man pointed to were *two goldfish* swimming in a bowl. That is how attitudes to sex have changed over the past twenty-five years.

One of the other changes is woman's liberation. How do you think it has affected men?

I don't think woman's liberation has been a good thing for men. Women who don't want, at least in part, to be sex objects are idiots—if they want to be thought of as one of the boys and not have a man fuck them. I think that any woman who wants to be one of the boys is either undersexed or unattractive. But I do understand and agree with women who don't want to be thought of as *just* sex objects. Of course, when a man sees a woman he still wants to take her to bed—not exclusively that, but he does sense that the woman is a sexual animal. I think that is a damn good thing. It is what keeps the race going and is something a woman should value.

How do you think a man should approach a woman he wants to go to bed with?

I think some men are afraid to approach a woman out of a fear of rejection. Of course jocks, football heros, who are used to women chasing them don't have a fear of rejection. I don't think I am an expert on how to approach a woman—I don't really know how to. But I do know that women are turned off if a man only wants them for sex. A woman who is bright and talented is not going to be turned on by a man who only wants to get her into bed. I think if you show a woman that you are interested in her as a person, then the sexual thing will follow. The way to approach a woman is as a human being. No lines—I think that is kind of old-hat. You have to treat a woman as a person. A lot of women are lonely; I've worked with most of the stars in the business and you'd be very surprised to discover how many famous women sit at home alone without a date. Men are afraid of them—they are afraid to call them.

How do you think a man can discover what kind of woman he has approached?

Very easy. He should talk to her—and more important, he should listen to her. Anyone will reveal himself or herself by just talking, so if you listen to what someone is saying, you will discover what kind of person she is. Discover what she is interested in, what she is all about. If that is difficult, if you feel you need clues, then you are with someone who is hiding. A lot of people hide behind masks, especially successful people. They feel they are not entitled to what they have; they are making millions of dollars a picture, they are invited to the White House, but deep inside they feel that they are ordinary; they remember their youth—they weren't born movie stars—and they feel they don't really deserve everything they have attained, that they are going to be found out one day. So they wear masks. A man falls in love with a woman who is famous and she feels, "If he finds out what I am really like he is not going to love me." So people who are unsure of themselves hide behind masks, hide behind an ideal they want to present to the world so that they will appear bright and talented, whereas inside they feel they are not.

On the subject of masks and faking, do you think you can recognize a woman's orgasm?

I think a woman who is a good actress can fake an orgasm so that there is no way that a man will be able to tell. There are some women who enjoy sex and don't have an orgasm, and don't even want one. But there are other women who feel that a climax is the final result of sex, and they want that pleasure. If a man doesn't bring that kind of woman to an orgasm then I think he should feel he has not been a satisfactory lover. I probably would feel a failure if I failed to bring a woman to a climax unless she told me it wasn't necessary.

You have been married for over twenty years—how do you keep romance and sexuality in such a long-term relationship?

You have to like the person you live with. It is hard to have sex with someone you don't care for. I think there should be variety in a sexual relationship. I don't care what turns you on—sometimes it is exciting to make love in different places, in different ways, or while you watch a porno movie. There has to be variation—and if either partner is uptight about sex it will become a problem, so that pretty soon the man or the woman will have to look for sex outside the relationship.

Do you think love and sex must always be related?

Not at all. But I think that is more true of men than of women. Of course there are women who are exceptions—women who will go to bed with a stranger because they like the look of his body or his face. But as a realistic generalization, women have the nest-building instinct, the children to take care of—while men don't have that responsibility, which is why men are not monogamous. A man can enjoy sex without love, but of course there is a difference in having sex with love and having sex without love. Without love, with a whore, or on a one-night-stand there is no continuity to sex. But if you are in love, then when the sex is over there is a wonderful feeling of fulfillment and sharing. You know you will share that with the woman again, you are building together. But if you have sex without love it is nothing—because it is a dead end.

What do you think makes a man good in bed?

Being interested in the woman and trying to please her. In sex, ninety percent of it is a woman trying to please a man in bed—and the other ninety percent is a man trying to please a woman in bed. Instead of being concerned about pleasing yourself, you should be concerned about pleasing your partner. That is what makes anyone good in bed—unselfishness.

Jan Murray

Like Sidney Sheldon, comedian Jan Murray, in his early sixties, has been married for over twenty years. His views present the values of family, fidelity, and Middle America. Jan Murray recalls a time when women weren't supposed to enjoy sex, when men went to $5 brothels, marriage was forever, and "people had far too many worries to spend too much time worrying about sex."

Zsa Zsa Gabor introduced me to Jan Murray during the taping of a TV show. I interviewed him a week later in his Hollywood Hills home, which Jan showed me before the interview began—the outdoor swimming pool, the view, his books on comedy, his awards, and most important of all, his family photographs. Jan explained that he had deliberately structured his life around home and family, knowing that success in show business is ephemeral: "The invitations are getting less, the bookings are also getting less, and more doors are closing. But I don't mind—I'm happy."

I have been married for over twenty-eight years—and when you have been married for that time you have to make love all day. In a sweet way, in a kind way, with a look, with a touch, with an embrace, a pet, a fondle, and a kindness. To make sex sweet and beautiful after twenty-eight years the preliminary work has to be done all day. I am not talking about bringing home presents or flowers—I have never done that. I don't have a big fight and then bring her home flowers—I try not to have the fight in the first place, and so does she. I do an act of kindness and my wife witnesses it—it turns her on about me. All of a sudden she is looking at me with such love. Kindness, an "I love you" during the course of the day, takes precedence over what happens in bed. It is very tough to be in the same bed seven nights a week and still be inventive and creative. The big creation is the turn-on. All that macho—all that sexuality in bed—is great for a while, but after that other things have to develop. What you do for each other out of bed keeps it fresh and new and beautiful. If you have been married for twenty-eight years you take the emphasis away from bed—bed is the culmination, the punchline, the curtain.

Sex has lost its mystery, its wonderment. When I grew up parents never discussed sex with children. I thought babies came out of foreheads till I was thirteen. I don't say that was the perfect way in which to be brought up, but I do think some beauty, some mystery, some mysticism, is good for sex. There is no way in the world that I would be interested in a woman if I knew somebody else had been there an hour ago. There would be no way I would want to be there too.

It was always hard for me to believe that some girls were loose and easy. At that time it was even hard for me to believe that girls had sexual desires the same as men. So I used to go out with girls that everyone else in the neighbourhood had had sex with—and I would just hold hands with them. I used to romance girls who were virtually hookers, and would never realize what they were. I always felt sex was sacred. Even if the girl had slept with lots of guys I believed that she was going out with me because she loved me and needed me and wanted me.

When I was fifteen I thought there was something wrong with me. The other guys were having erections, and sex and all that, but I wasn't. I was having erections in my house—but I hadn't had sex. The guys bullied me about it, and one day cornered me and dragged me to a whorehouse in the Bronx. We went for five dollars—she was a poor, ugly girl in a robe, broken-down, terrible. I went into her room and I couldn't do it. I gave her a dollar tip, told her to tell the other guys I was with that it was great, talked to her for ten minutes, got dressed, went outside to the other guys, and said it was terrific.

I was finally introduced to sex by a married woman. I was a young comedian of sixteen, working in the Catskills for three dollars a week. She was a beautiful woman and she helped promulgate my romantic vision of sex. In order to assuage her own guilt feelings—to justify cheating on her husband—she made the experience a romantic, beautiful thing, for herself and for me. But then I met her husband, who was one of the nicest guys I'd ever met in my life, and from that day on there was no way I could have sex with a woman if I knew her husband. I was always a romantic, dreamed of romantic things, and thought romantic thoughts with girls. Growing up in the Depression, worried about food and shelter, I had too many worries to spend too much time worrying about sex. Nowadays people have very few worries, so instead they worry about sex.

It is difficult nowadays to shock me about anything. I go out on stage every night for an hour to make people laugh—so I have to know what is going on in the world. But even today if I tell a dirty joke in front of ladies I find myself apologizing. At a private function I might say, "Look, I have to use one or two dirty words." Sometimes the women say, "Fine." Sometimes I can see they are reluctant, so I don't use as strong a joke as I was going to. But I think the language of love should be different from street language. When I am arguing with a guy I might tell him to "Go fuck himself," so then it is hard for me to use that word with somebody I love in a moment of tender passion.

I am often at conventions for groups of guys. I don't give a damn whether the guys are cab drivers, lawyers, professors, truck drivers, or judges, but if you put ten guys in a room the conversation immediately turns to sex and dames, who you can call and what you can do with them. I would suggest that a lot of married guys instead of getting involved somewhere would be better off if they paid a hundred dollars and got themselves a lovely girl who knows where it's at. Personally I believe that you need a companion, somebody who has lived a whole life with you. I suppose I could have lived with some dame for ten years, then another one, then another one—that might have had its own excitement, I suppose. But nothing could replace the ultimate happiness of my life with my wife, my children, and my grandchildren—my life and my family.

Huntington Hartford

Multimillionaire A&P heir and philanthropist Huntington Hartford lives in a different world from Jan Murray. High above New York's plush Beekman Place, lonely because his wife was away at the time, Huntington Hartford seemed like a guest in his own house, surrounded by servants who constantly followed him around. I arrived at five in the afternoon to find Huntington Hartford in a beige robe, eating his breakfast of mashed-up boiled egg out of a bowl. While he ate, I waited in another room with Jackie Hartford, his son, a student at Juilliard. For a while we watched *The Longest Day* on television. A plaster ornament, proclaiming "The Biggest Sportsman in the World," sat on top of the TV. Huntington Hartford appeared and disappeared at intervals without saying a word to me.

I had begun to feel like an inferior piece of furniture, and to doubt that an interview would be forthcoming, when I was finally summoned into the next room. The room was elegant, filled with paintings and photographs of Huntington Hartford with President Kennedy and other notable public figures. I turned the tape recorder on, dubious about the response. I needn't have worried; the moment the switch clicked Huntington Hartford also switched on, instantly becoming the ideal interviewee.

His attitude toward sex is a curious mixture of modern and old-fashioned. He says he likes women to do unusual things in bed, but at the same time believes sex is of secondary importance to a woman. I was also interested in the interview's other topics—Huntington Hartford's business failures, his insecurity, his comments on model agencies, and the details about his wives.

I have worried about being good in bed because I don't think I am particularly good. I think that to a great extent, being good in bed is endowment, and men are either born with that or they aren't. A great lover is usually well endowed physically and able to come three or four times in one night—I don't happen to fall into that category. I also don't have a great deal of vitality—so far as sex goes, I am not the ideal lover. But I do have certain qualifications for being good in bed. I understand women well—I've always understood them in a way, and that usually grows as you get older. I really didn't know what sex was about until my thirties. I think the average guy is immature in his twenties—and that the best sexual ages of men are the thirties, forties, and fifties. I think the most important thing is to be a *man*—because if a man is attractive, sincere, and understanding and really appeals to a woman, in the sense that he does what she wants, a woman will forgive a lot of failings in sex.

I suppose women made me feel inadequate—probably because of an inferiority complex on my part. I was always shy, but I am attracted to my opposite—to experienced, boyish-looking, sophisticated girls. In a way, I think New York is unfortunate so far as women are concerned because the model agencies there have tremendous power, and a great deal is controlled by them. The opinions of Wilhelmina and Ford have a great deal to do with the attitudes of young girls to men. To some extent the model agencies get into the private lives of the girls and control them.

I don't think women's lib has changed the relationship between men and women, because sexual attitudes are instinctive. The most important thing is if a girl is attracted to a man and likes him. I never worried whether a woman wanted me for myself or for my

money. The problem is how to handle money—how to
preserve it and to use it well. Unfortunately, when I in-
herited my grandfather's trust in 1957, I didn't know
how to handle money. I lost a lot in the early
1960s—I had no business adviser at all except my
lawyers, and I don't think they handled it as I should
have. If a man knows how to handle money, then I
think the right woman will come to him.

I think sex should be an equal relationship; I don't
think it matters who the initiator is. Although I do
think that the best situation is when the man talks the
woman into bed—or at least *thinks* he does. I think a
man should ask for what he wants in bed, if he thinks
the woman will do it. If a woman wants to do something unusual in bed, and I'm attracted to her,
great!—I am delighted.

I think going to bed is secondary to a woman, even
though it may be foremost in a man's mind. I think the
pleasure men and women get from sex is quite different; a man comes several times and a woman comes
relatively few times. But I don't think orgasm is the
most important thing in the world. It *is* important, but
it's not the ideal answer to the relationship between a
man and a woman. I don't think it matters that much
if a woman fakes orgasm—everything depends on her
attitude to me. It's all right if a woman fakes because
she cares about me, because she is having a good time
and I appeal to her.

I think the men who really appeal to women—are
successful in the right kind of way, know how to be
gentlemen—but have a little macho in them, are touch
guys like the Sicilians. I admire the Sicilians' ability to
have so much vitality and to be so involved in life. I
don't think I have it nearly as much as they do. Sicilians are good storytellers, charming, touch, with a certain flamboyance, and are good in bed. I don't think
Sicilians care much about women—they care about the
relationship between men as friends, and they like girls
who sit quietly in the background. That's not what I

want. My wife calls these people "street people"—and I think it's true. She happens to like street people—I don't think she really understands me—but I don't really like to go into it.

I grew up in a very sheltered way and I was very shy. My father died when I was twelve, and I was very much under the domination of my mother. So one of the reasons for my first marriage was to be freer. Then I fell in love with Marjorie—my second wife—who was the great, great love of my life. She is one of the few geniuses I've ever known. I got her interested in art when she was about eighteen, and she did all the paintings in my apartment. I was married to Marjorie for twelve years. At that time she had a bit of a drinking problem, which she has since completely overcome. I was on my own to a great extent, and we just got separated for a long time. Then she fell in love with a deep-sea diver and I was extremely upset. I was married to my third wife, Diane, for seven years, and had a little daughter, Juliet. I think that marriage wasn't the best thing I could have done at that time. Then I was single till 1970, when I married my present wife—I was very attracted to her.

The best thing of all is if you are really in love with someone. But I think it's extremely rare to find a love that is physically, mentally, emotionally, and financially right. And I also think friendship is very important. There is a story about Somerset Maugham. His mother and father were called Beauty and the Beast; his mother was so beautiful and his father was so ugly. Someone once asked Mrs. Maugham why she loved such an ugly man. And I've never forgotten her answer: "Because he never hurts my feelings." If I had to live my life over again—there are many things I would have done differently. I have a lot of regrets.

Rod Steiger

ROD STEIGER: Tell me the difference between a man you would go to bed with and one you wouldn't. (I'm getting a marvelous interview!)

WENDY: *I wouldn't go to bed with someone unsubtle.*

ROD STEIGER: Too direct?

WENDY: *No—that sometimes turns me on. By unsubtlety I mean making a clumsy first approach, not watching my reactions, and not trying to discover what I am like—what I like.*

ROD STEIGER: Did you have a bad experience in America?

WENDY: *I found many American men didn't know how to initiate a relationship—they just gave me a routine and didn't play the moment.*

ROD STEIGER: Define "play the moment."

WENDY: *I try to play the moment in a relationship by not having the same expectations I had from the last relationship, not doing or saying the same things, or being the same fixed person. In an interview I try to play the moment by not having a fixed formula, not knowing in advance what I want to find, not sticking to a rigid list of questions.*

Perhaps I should have had a list of questions when I went to interview Rod Steiger, because I ended up *being* interviewed, losing control of the interview, confronted by a barrage of questions. As Rod says himself, he would have made a great DA, and at times the experience was unnerving. I found myself forced to define my definitions, qualify my statements, explain my prejudices, and analyze my intentions. I felt momentarily flattered by Rod Steiger's apparent interest in my mind and opinions—until retrospectively I realized that I was probably just a testing ground for his own very formulated ideas on love, sex, and relationships. Those ideas are partly the product of years of therapy and Steiger's own work with patients in a California clinic. The interview reflects Rod Steiger's strong self-searching quality.

I interviewed Rod Steiger in his suite at the Savoy Hotel, London, where he was visiting his teenage daughter by his marriage to Clare Bloom. The British press was full of stories about Steiger's pending vitriolic third divorce, so when I phoned for an interview I expected gruffness and was pleasantly surprised when he agreed to see me. When I arrived, Rod was polite, offered me a drink, answered the phone continuously—till we started talking. He held all calls, we spoke for two hours, then Steiger left for dinner, protesting about having to wear a tie.

A few days later we met again and I showed him the text. Rod read it carefully, with extreme caution, pausing only to correct my spelling. At that moment he sounded like a cross between a schoolmaster and W.C. Fields—my favorite of all Steiger's film portrayals. In many ways, Rod Steiger was also one of my favorite interviewees; tremendously articulate, very focused, sharper than most critics, sometimes gregarious, other times taciturn, often autocratic, occasionally patronizing, always attractive.

Do you think you have changed a great deal sexually since you grew up?

I have to question "grew up"—because I don't think I've grown up that much. And I don't think I should.

The essence of creativity in a human being comes from
the childish forces within us, which are also in conflict
with the parental and adult forces within. I wouldn't
want to sacrifice the childish forces in me—because
even though they hurt me a great deal, by making me
lose my temper and making me feel sorry for myself,
they are still the foundation out of which you get crazy
impulses which lead to discoveries in art and in relationships.

*How does that apply to your relationships with
women?*

There is definitely a connection between the childish
and the romantic. My childish impulses led me to one
of the loveliest women I have ever known. I saw her at
the Caprice Restaurant in London, sitting at a table
with a group of people. Had I been completely adult I
would have tried to memorize her as a pleasant
memory to carry around in my life. But we exchanged
looks—and the childish part of me ignited the romantic. I happen to be pretty good at sketching, so I
sketched her and in an infantile creative way sent the
sketch over to her table. She smiled at me, and I fig-
ured that was the end of that. I began to feel a little
sad at the end of what might have been an interesting
relationship. I watched her across the room—then suddenly she came over, said hello, and introduced herself.
So the childish became the romantic and led to the
creative, which in turn led to love.

*I've told you how I feel about the initial approach of
many men. How would you advise them to approach a
woman?*

Any man who asks a woman to make love to him is
an idiot. You don't wait for a woman to say yes. I've
never said to a woman, "Will you fuck me?" and then
waited for a yes. It's a matter of vibrations, and I don't
believe I can define vibrations. If I could I'd be King

Solomon and King Kong put together. (I'd rather be Solomon. I went through my King Kong phase.) And if I knew I wouldn't be in the middle of my third divorce. It's all the clichés—something happens—a look in the eyes—a connection—a touch of the hands —why does one skin feel better than the other? You just exchange looks. Once the woman's eye has given you permission—and she doesn't *tell* you—you feel it. Only then can you really go to bed with that woman— because you can't very well enjoy the company of a woman in bed if she doesn't want to be there. Unless you knock her out, in which case she is not going to be very exciting.

How do you think a man can find out what a woman wants in bed?

The greatest admissions are made in silence. It has to do with the look in the eyes—with vibrations, with imagination. You must stop being so verbal.

The only reasons I am being so verbal and concentrating on that approach are that men often make clumsy verbal approaches and that both men and women have told me that they want to talk to their partner about their sexual desires but find it difficult.

If a woman wants something from a man or vice-versa, I would say; don't ask them, don't leave them, just start to do it—and if he or she doesn't want to they have a right to say yes or no—or certainly discuss it. The trouble is that both sexes have the tendency to put each other on a pedestal. Women think, "Well, if I ask him to kiss the left cheek of my ass, he is going to think that I am terrible." The religions of the world have taught us that we are not supposed to do certain things with someone we love—but that it's all right to go out and do them with someone you don't love. Bullshit. Work it out together, so that the understanding between the two of you becomes deeper and greater.

Go and do whatever you can think of with someone you love, and you've got a good thing going.

Do you think love is essential to sex?

No. It is very important not to confuse love with sex or with curiosity. Curiosity has put more people into bed than romance. Although perhaps love may be the continuation of curiosity. The first thing that happens to you when you walk into a room is you talk to a woman you are curious about—a human being who is appealing to you. Intelligence is very important to me in a woman, so if I go over to a woman and she talks with no brain, I can make up my mind and say, Well, I am not here for brains, but I am here for a little sport loving, so I will have my sport love for that evening. That will then be what is coldly called a one-night stand—but on the other hand if I walk over to that woman and we happen to have the same interests in common, you may have the beginning of a romance.

A romance may last three days, it may last three years, it may last thirty years. There is no telling—and there shouldn't be; there should never be a time limit on the length of a romance. In my way of acting I believe that you enter into the moment and you go wherever it takes you, trying at the same time to be as honest as possible—then you may discover something worthwhile. The same applies to relationships. When I start a relationship I don't know exactly what is going to happen except that if I present myself completely honestly as I am there is a possibility that I will get back a more complete response from somebody else who is also trying to be more themselves by participation in life, with life, through me.

Does anything shock you sexually?

There is only so much you can do in bed. It's how one does it. The man is going to enter the woman's body, and she is going to give her body to him. Then there is oral sex and all sorts of games you can play leading up to sex—wherever heightens it for each other. I have a motto—a joke—I say, "Anything goes in the bedroom except real blood." Or real pain—or real fear. Pretending to be afraid, pretending to be in pain, could be part of the fun of it. But I don't want any whips laid on my back, and if there is a mark there that lasts any time or blood, it's time for me to say goodbye. Otherwise there are no rules—just no pain, and no lying. Fantasies are very important, depending on the day and on your mood. I'd be very happy to be a slave, I'd be very happy to be a master, I'd be very happy to play a priest, I'd be very happy to play policeman, and I don't care as long as it is enjoyable. If I am out for a good time—there are other times when if there are any other women present; as long as I am the only man, that's fine with me. That doesn't necessarily mean, though, that my prowess is going to satisfy them all. But it certainly doesn't matter if you feel that way once in a while.

Did you ever worry about sex when you were growing up?

Yes, I did. I think the first worry—the first thing young men did, was to compare the size of their cocks. That led to exhibiting them to each other and seeing if one could urinate farther than the other. Then mutual masturbation, till we became fascinated by the miracle of an orgasm. And that was the beginning of worry—which later on made us think something was wrong with ourselves. Then we realized everybody did that, so we all felt better. We were very like little groups of animals, fondling themselves, playing with themselves, and enjoying themselves. Most men go through the rest of their lives doing that. So you went through the beginning of normal development and the next thing was getting interested in the opposite sex and getting worried about how you could get to them.

Do you think men masturbate as much as women?

I think they are pretty even. There are some women that don't and there are some men that don't—so I am sure the mastabatory habits of males and females equal out. Nature is too smart not to keep a balance. Nature has no favorites. I discovered that when they were wheeling me down the hall of the hospital and I had to have four veins put into my heart. It gave me a shock, took me off Mount Olympus, and said; "You see, my friend, you are not a god."

If nature makes everything sexual equal, are there any rules?

No rules. The thing about love and sex that is so incredible is that they are like life—which I choose to spell flux. A state of constant change. It's the way the day goes, the way the animal in you changes, that determines the kind of love you will make that particular day. Example: Exhausted partner comes home. Exhausted partner should be put on top at the beginning. But you will find out that before it's over, the one on the bottom will be on top or sideways, or whatever. So much depends on what kind of a day you've had. There are times when you make love quickly—you are through the door and you are bending over a chair or on the floor—and you haven't even taken your clothes off. Then there are other times when both of you do everything you can think of—the cologne, the incense, a little grass, everything—but it's still a number-one disaster. There are times that you make love for thirty seconds—but it's worth thirty years—there are other times when you've made love for thirty years and it isn't even worth thirty seconds.

What advice would you give a man about being good in bed?

A man who doesn't acknowledge the feminine part

of his makeup will never be good in the bedroom. There is a feminine side and a masculine side to each sex. And in bed a man can be a father to a woman, or like a mother to her. You have to learn when to move and when not to move and when to play what through experience, intelligence, and imagination. You either have it or you don't, and if you don't have imagination you will never be good at fantasies. But you can't make an unimaginative partner imaginative. I've tried that— forget it. You have to realize that the bedroom is not a place for fucking, it is a place to make into a form of paradise in any way you can. The bedroom must be and must always remain a land of fantasy. It is not a church or a cathedral or a synagogue or a Buddhist temple but a playroom, a playground where you go to play. Technique can be taught, and two people can be equal in technique—but not in talent or imagination. Being good in bed is instinct and technique, imagination, talent, and living enough to gather an education out of the pain of your experiences. Then applying the new facts you found through those particular experiences. Put all that together with sexual drive and you are going to have one hell of a man walking into that bedroom.

Barry Newman

Television star Barry Newman agrees with Richard Burton that men are born sexual. But unlike Burton, he is very much a product of the '50s. Newman typifies the macho man many of the experts talked about in the beginning of the book. He admits that intellectually he understands female liberation, but that emotionally he is "still of the school that believes a man can screw anything that walks, but that a woman belongs in the

kitchen." A self-confessed chauvinist, Barry
Newman's attitude to sex and women isn't
clouded by professions of equality or enlightened
remarks like "I only want an intelligent
woman"—which in practice men don't always
truly mean. I disagree with Barry Newman's as-
sumptions, but I appreciate his honesty. In the interview he has the courage to flaunt his
male-chauvinist convictions, and the confidence
born of being an eligible Beverly Hills bachelor.

I phoned Barry Newman from New York, his
service took my message, and two days later
Barry phoned from L.A.—rare for a celebrity to
return a call. I told him about my book. He kept
calling me "sweetheart" and sounded slightly like
Bogart. Once in Los Angeles, I interviewed Barry
Newman in his apartment. As a new arrival, I was
unprepared for the heat, felt sweaty, and wanted
to regain my "English rose" cool. Barry suggested
I put on his dark-green silk robe. I did and we
talked—while the phone rang incessantly, with a
different "sweetheart" calling each time. I con-
cluded that I was talking to Warren Beatty's
clone; I became uneasy and felt compromised by
just wearing the green silk robe. However, Barry
was enthusiastic about the topic, always polite,
very much the respectful "older brother."

I love sex—and I think a woman should be thrilled
if I am making love to her. I think women are here to
give a man pleasure. I like to give pleasure too—there
are very few great cocksmen in the world. I have had
twenty-one years of going out with girls—I've had so
much experience—and experience makes you confident.

But I was a very slow starter. In the '50s guys all
wanted to "score"—to score was really something. You
would say things like "How did you do?" or "I got a
bare tit" or "You mean you really got her bra off?"

You really worked at scoring. Then suddenly it was the '60s—very casual—you watched all those young kids who weren't interested in scoring; if it happened, it happened.

All my friends already fooled around when they were fourteen, but I was a really shy, twitchy kid and couldn't get a girl. When I was seventeen I went to play the saxophone with a group and I didn't have to be aggressive or assertive any more because as I was a musician the girls all came on to me. My first sexual experience was at seventeen, with a girl who was a senior in high school. I didn't know whether I was good or bad—I would reach a climax in about ten seconds. But in time I acquired a sense of control. Apart from that, sex is instructive. Some men are more passionate than others, some men naturally know how to touch.

I know I can walk up to a woman in the street, pinch her ass within three minutes—and she'll smile. If nine other guys did the same thing, she would slap their faces. I can be inside a woman within five minutes of meeting her and she'll say, "Isn't he adorable?" whereas with nine other men she will be shouting, "Rape!" I never ask a woman to go to bed with me—I would never say, "Will you go to bed with me?" —because even if the woman is the biggest whore in the world she is going to say, "Of course not." If I am attracted to a woman I tell her so, but I think a man should be like a hawk: come in for the kill, then move back, always move back. Some men just say, "Come back to my apartment," and three minutes later, grab the woman. It rarely works. A girl should always be made to feel comfortable, because if she is comfortable then she will trust the man.

The trouble with most men is that they are too fast. You should be very slow—you should warm the woman up. If you warm her up to the point of no return, before you enter her, that is what she wants. I know from experience what a woman wants; she wants to be toyed with, to reach a plateau, so she can't turn back or stop herself. A man has got to know how to touch a woman, beautifully and gently, how to touch her so there's no return. When I started having sex, a piano player named Joey Masters—the make-out king of Boston—told me never to forget that the clitoris is the most sensitive part of a woman. "Remember," he said, "there isn't a woman alive who doesn't love to be eaten." And I said, "You must be kidding."

You can always feel the orgasm if you are passionate. I can't tell if a woman fakes in bed—my ego is so big, I never imagine a woman would need to fake with me. You will always find something that works with every woman if you try lots of different things with her. I found that the majority of women like to be talked to in bed. I love all women to talk in bed—that is a great turn-on. I can't stand silence in bed, just as I can't stand darkness. I always discuss the sex with the woman afterward—not before, because if you start an intellectual conversation up front it destroys the romance. I find that women are much more uninhibited than men but they are afraid to show it. They want to be led—they are afraid that if the man sees their lack of inhibitions he will be shocked. So a man has to know how to be very open, to lead the conversation and show the woman what he likes. I believe the man is the dominant force (I guess I'm chauvinistic in my attitude to women).

I have refused things a woman has asked me to do to her in bed because I didn't like the way in which she asked. If a woman I am in bed with suddenly says, "Do this," "Do that," "A little bit to the left," "A little bit to the right," then I say, "This girl is a traffic cop."

Once a woman made me feel sexually inadequate, and I'll never forget it. I was impotent with that woman because right in the middle she said, "I am not feeling your love—don't you understand?—I am not feeling your passion." It ruined the whole thing. Also, sometimes I've been with the same woman for a month and suddenly haven't had an erection with her for a week. I felt strange because I could walk along the street, see something new, and have an erection immediately. I felt badly for the girl but I didn't worry about it myself. It's something that happens to men now and then and even happened to me occasionally in my early twenties. But I usually get bored by sameness in bed.

I had as many pretty girls when I was starting out in show business as I do now. There are a lot of men who want to have a gorgeous girl on their arm, a sex symbol, an image, but then they can't get it up. Most guys try to have the image of a cocksman—but they know that we know that most of them are not really cocksmen. Although there *are* some guys who get laid three times a day with four different women. A woman once told me that she had had an affair with a famous lover but he was the worst lover in the world. Whereas, I think, the guy had probably had fifteen minutes, the girl had come in, he had just wanted to get off and forget all about her. He was just interested in getting his rocks off and not in being great in bed.

I have felt the pressure to be great in bed. Sometimes I've had the pressure of feeling I've had to sleep with a woman when I didn't want to. I had started necking with her when suddenly she got very passionate. And I've had to play the feminine role and say, "I'm tired," or "I've got to leave." And I felt guilty. Also—and a lot of married men feel this pressure—if you have been seeing a girl for a long time, sometimes you want to sleep, but then she feels rejected, and that you haven't been paying enough attention to her, so you have the pressure to perform. Those are the only sexual pressures I have felt. I don't have a complex about the size of my penis or anything like that. I know when you talk to a woman she will say, "It's not the size—it's how you use it." But in actuality when women are together they say, "He had one that big."

I am still of the school that believes that a man can screw anything that walks, but that a woman belongs in the kitchen. That women should be waiting by the phone for me to call them. Intellectually I know that is not what is happening, but most men are afraid to admit that this is actually what they would like to see. And so many men are impotent nowadays because they feel they have to be good lovers. Whereas I feel, "Let the girl satisfy me." Lee Strasberg used to say, "Acting is reacting." That is a wonderful lesson for being good in bed. The man could be the greatest lover in the world, but if the woman is not reacting then the sex is useless.

John Newcombe

When I asked Australian tennis star John Newcombe for an interview, he roared with laughter—and then talked to me for half an hour. We sat by the pool at Caesar's Palace in Las Vegas, where John was competing in Johnny Carson's tennis tournament. Muscular, suntanned, with aquamarine eyes, John Newcombe rivals any cigarette-ad male model. During the interview, John drank beer. John sometimes makes fun of his Australian image and at one point laughingly confessed that all Australian men really want is a lot of mates, a lot of beer, and an occasional Sheila.

John Newcombe's interview takes a backward glance at sex in America and Australia during the 1950s. Like Barry Newman, Jim Brown, and Jan Murray, John recalls teenage bragging about sexual prowess. Like Rod Steiger, he believes a woman can and should initiate a relationship. And like Huntington Hartford, John Newcombe thinks that having an orgasm is secondary to a woman.

I have been married for eleven years, and most of the other guys on the tennis circuit are also now married. The bachelors on the circuit had varying types of relationships with women. There was the girl you met for the night and went home with, probably for just a one-night affair. In that kind of affair it depended on the woman whether the relationship stayed as a bang-bang relationship or whether the man felt he had to prove himself to be a fantastic lover. But with tennis groupies sex was usually a selfish act for both of you.

Sex has changed since I was a bachelor, because then women didn't have the Pill and didn't feel so free; they were afraid of getting pregnant and held back. Before about 1967, American women were the least likely to go to bed with a man. Today they are probably more likely to than any other nationality, because I think they have achieved a liberation of their feelings. The Pill has taken away all the scares.

I think that women control sex much more than men do. If the woman is too passive then the man finds it hard to get mentally stimulated. If she's too aggressive then it's hard for the man to get emotionally stimulated. The woman has to achieve something in between. I also think it is easier for women than for men to have sex. A woman probably enjoys sex even if she doesn't have an orgasm, but if a man feels pressured to make a woman come then he won't enjoy the sex. Some women don't reach orgasm very quickly, so then the pressure is on the man to help her, to perform.

When you have been married for eleven years, you develop the relationship to the point where you are not obliged to prove yourself the greatest lover in the world every time you go to bed with your wife. Sometimes it's good, sometimes it's very good, sometimes it's terrific. I can't remember it ever being bad. It's a matter of not worrying about sex or feeling it has to be an almighty affair every time you go to bed.

I worried about being good in bed when I was about fifteen, because at that time everyone at school was telling stories about sex, everyone was bragging. Probably about ninety per cent of us were lying about how we did in bed, because I'm sure most fellows of that age have doubts about whether they are doing a good job. I will tell my son that it is very important that he learn about sex—all about his body, and a woman's body—so that he will understand sex. Also he will then have less chance of getting her pregnant. I'd probably also give him a few books to read, and advise him to be open and honest in his relationship and never take advantage of a woman. Nowadays boys seem to start sex at fifteen—and I know my son will get caught by a girl about that age. I say "caught" because I think men go out for the night, notice a girl, and think, "I'm going to get her," but in reality the girl is probably already marking him the moment he walks into the room. If a girl wants a guy, she'll get him. Whereas if a guy sees a girl, he won't automatically get her. But a girl can get any guy she wants to—if she is attractive she can play any game she wants.

I don't imagine that the fact I am a sportsman and in good condition makes me better in bed. I don't think stamina and staying power have anything to do with being good in bed. The buildup before going to bed is just as important as anything, because the thought and mental feeling has to be there to make it a nicer, more lasting affair. For most women the most important thing is to feel tenderness, and loving and care. The approach has to open and honest. To me sex is really another form of conversation between two people; it's another way of talking but with actions. Letting your feelings out without words.

Jim Brown

I was warned about you—people told me to be careful. Something about you throwing a girl out of a window?

I'm no sadistic cat.

I never did discover the details of that story. All I do know is that Jim Brown confounded my expectations. I had imagined him big, tall, and brutal. Instead he wasn't very tall, not particularly broad-shouldered, and appeared attentive and gentle. We sat on the terrace of his house overlooking Sunset Boulevard. At first I was too hot, so Jim spent a long time moving around the sun umbrella to give me shade. The interview lasted an hour and twenty minutes, with Jim answering quickly and emphatically. At the end of the interview he signed a release form. I asked if I could use his frank remark about Tom Jones, and Jim said, "Yes. It's the truth. I don't want to hurt his feelings, but it's the truth."

Jim Brown's interview could aptly be subtitled "Beyond Barry Newman." I had heard Hollywood stories of his youthful wildness (Jim Brown himself says, "Guys go through a certain stage of life when they want to get some pussy"), but Jim seems to have emerged into maturity secure, concerned now about love and relationships as well as sex. "You realize that living isn't about performance or nonperformance," he said. I initially asked him about the problems of having a super-stud sportsman image—but I felt chastened by his response: "My life is absolutely the opposite of what people think, the women, the sex, the foot-

ball. My aim for the past sixteen years has been
social change and equality for blacks. We have
started education programs for dropouts—we
were down at Marshall County, Mississippi, to get
people food and medical supplies, trying to entice
industry to move in so there would be jobs. Right
now we are waiting for Washington to give us
some help—if we raise one million, the govern-
ment will give us four million in order to allow
minorities to get into big business. If we are able
to get this we will make films that aren't degrading, with a different emphasis on black participation. That is where my head is really at—it's
where my head has always been, and I'm not saying that to impress anyone."

I am not Superman—neither is anyone else—so why
should I pretend? When I was a kid all I heard about
sex was performance—how quickly you could get a
woman, how many women you'd got, what you did to
a woman, how long you did it to her, how well you did
it, and how great in bed you were. Sex was always doing something *to* a woman, never doing something *with*
her. Consequently you wondered about yourself, if you
were not doing that, if you liked this, if you weren't
making love to a woman for five hours in a row. Sex
was turned into a test—something you were great at, if
you did it well.

Our society approaches sex from the standpoint of a
lie. Everything one is taught or hears about sex is from
an exaggerated point of view. Sex is not as good as
people say, and it's not as bad as people say. It's in the
middle, and it's never been put into its proper perspec-
tive. Everybody has weaknesses and strengths.

Many people are insecure about sex—and I'm the
same as anybody else, I've gone through the same
things, except I've learned and as I became a man
found my own values. Even though you may feel insecure for a while, you quickly get out of that and begin

dealing with individual women. You realize that living isn't about performance or nonperformance—it's really about caring for someone and having someone care about you. Deep down inside most of my friends feel that way too, but they don't express it because of a macho type of attitude. Of course guys go through a certain stage of life when they want to get some pussy, as they say, but deep down most men would prefer to have a good woman—a woman that makes them happy and that they make happy. That's difficult to find.

I like sex—I'm a physical lover. But I never dealt with trying to get one-night stands. Even though I might make love to a woman on the first night, I always dealt with her as a human being. She could always see me again or talk to me again. I don't think you have to be in love to make love, but I do think sex with the woman you love has got to be the best sex you've had. Relationships have always been more important to me than sex. My first girlfriend played the role of girlfriend, and family. So I don't separate the two. I think about loyalty, about who cares for me, about who will look out for me.

I've had beautiful girlfriends, I've had intelligent girlfriends. I've got a beautiful, intelligent girl now. She's got a nice mother and father and she likes me. When I first saw her I liked the way she looked and I told her. Then I told her I didn't have time for long courtships—which was a line out of a movie I produced. She thought I just wanted to make love to her—but I was playing. I had patience with her—I found out that she was very intelligent, that she was worth having patience with. I didn't entice her with any false promises, but told her where I wanted to get. I was very natural and honest with her, because that is the only way I can reach the kind of relationship I want with a woman.

No two women are ever the same—you have to deal with them on vibrations. There are some women whom you don't have to say anything to, and they know you like them. But there are other women to whom you could say anything in the world and they would never like you. I can look at a woman and know if I like her physically. It's a combination of her personality and what she is physically. Maybe she's funny, maybe she's cute, maybe she's aloof—there are a lot of things I might like.

Every woman is different. People talk about "what you want sexually" and "what I want sexually," but that is assuming that all people know what they want. A woman can show me something that I've never seen—and it can be fantastic, something that happens in a moment. A woman can arrive at what she likes sexually with an individual man, but that same thing may not work with another man. Maybe she likes having her toes sucked by one man, but having them sucked by another man may not make any difference. The main thing a man should do is respond to what he is dealing with—to give and to take. Sometimes I look at a woman and I see something in her—and instead of planning everything in a relationship and saying "I like that" and the woman saying "I like this" and then doing it, you should let things happen.

Great sex is what makes you feel good. It's when I can satisfy my woman and feel her satisfaction and then in turn be satisfied. I don't think you can just be good in bed in general, with everybody. If you go around trying to make love to everybody there are going to be a lot of failures. The thing is to try to find out what is—not what is supposed to be.

I never felt that I had to live up to a sexy image. There are so many different images of me: the football player, the movie actor, the locker-room lawyer, the brutal guy who likes to fight. There are women who want to make love with a man because of his image—because he is a sportsman. I never had much of a problem with that because I've always insisted on being an individual all my life. I am a man—my occupation has nothing to do with what I am. When people thought of me as a sportsman it had nothing to do with me. I always thought that being a sportsman was like being an overrated gladiator—like being in a zoo.

I'm a truthful person, and they can't take that away. I had the chance of being the all-American boy—of becoming a Mark Spitz or an O. J. Simpson. All I had to do was what they told me to do. But I just did not think any amount of money was worth having an image where you take orders from other people as to what is best for that image. In that situation I could never have spoken about race, I could never have spoken out about equality for all men, I could never have done all the things that I do. Deep in my heart I feel that anyone who allows himself to be commercialized to the point where he can never make a public statement that is not monitored is less than a man. I am free.

Jim Brown is no different from any other man in the world. Although I might have had the opportunity to love some very beautiful ladies—I've made movies with Raquel Welch, Jackie Bisset, Brenda Sykes—some of the most beautiful ladies in the world. To all the men in the world: you haven't missed a thing. Because you can't make love to an image. Working with Racquel Welch is good to tell somebody about—but if you don't get on with her, it's no good. Sex is a one-to-one situation, and if you find a lady who cares about you—and who you care about—then you are living as good as any man in the world.

Andy Warhol

Andy Warhol's interview is an interlude—a space between interviews, which the uninitiated might call spacy. Segments of me reacted contrastingly to Andy Warhol. One segment was puzzled, another impressed, another intimidated, another admiring of Marilyn and pop art, another bewildered—while the rest of me liked him, realizing simultaneously that I probably needed an interpreter.

With his name enshrined daily in print, Andy Warhol is hard-core chic to *le tout* Paris, *le tout* Londres, *le tout* New York, not to mention *le monde entier*. Instantly recognizable, unimpeachably fashionable, Andy Warhol's name has become a brand name, a beacon borne by every socialite and social climber. Naturally, only his first name is necessary—Andy as in Liza, Margaux, Marisa, Bianca, and Regine.

I first met Andy Warhol at Regine's in Paris, where I was introduced to him by the incomparably beautiful Dewi Sukarno. With unblinking determination, Andy snapped his Polaroid at everyone. He was undeniably the focal point of the evening. I met him again at Regine's in New York, minus Polaroid, but intently watching the colorful scene from the side.

Later that month I talked to Andy Warhol in the frantic atmosphere of his New York office, while Liza's secretary called on one line, Halston on the other. After the interview we gossiped in a friendly way (but would he recognize me in the street? can I even *imagine* him in the street?). Then I left. A few months later, after seeing Andy at more parties, always the inscrutable star, I went back to his office, where he wordlessly signed the release. So here is Andy Warhol, enigma, artist, international superstar, on another way of sex.

You know a lot of glamorous women—what do you think they are looking for in a man?

I never see any of them find anything. I've only been

to one marriage and that was Marisa's. I don't know anyone who married except Marisa. Most of the girls I know are actually looking for work—and they are looking for men who can get them movie parts.

What advice would you give to a man who wants to be good in bed?

Just get there.

Would you rather watch people have sex—or have it yourself?

If the people were really young and beautiful I'd rather watch. I think if people really *have* to have sex, they should stop when they are twenty-two. I think anyone over twenty-two—old people—are ugly doing it.

What do you think of sex clubs like Plato's Retreat?

I think they are a great idea. I know lots of people who go to Plato's Retreat—but it should only be for young people.

You've made films in which people have sex. What do you think of sex on film?

In the movies they make sex look better than it is. They take a week to film each scene—so sex looks better on film than it is when you do it for real. But when I saw the film *Three Women* there were old people doing it and it really turned me off.

Who do you think is more driven by sex—men or women?

They are driven equally.

Who do you think has more complexes about sex—men or women?

I think they both have the same amount of complexes. Women worry about not having big breasts. And men worry about not having big penises. But if you look at a statue of a nude man it actually looks better when it is small. I've been doing some painting, so I see a lot—and when they are really big they look terrible.

If you could create an ideal sexual world, what would it be like?

I think taking a pill instead of having sex would be more exciting.

Whom do you fantasize about?

No one.

Can you describe your ideal sex partner?

My dog.

And . . .

Snow White. Pure. And she didn't have big breasts. I guess I like girls who have brand names. Like Katherine Guinness. Names have sex appeal. Heinz, Bloomingdale's, Bendel's, Ford's. I usually see a dollar sign on the person's forehead. Money is more important than having a big cock. Sex is overrated.

People say you are asexual. What does that mean to you?

I just don't think about sex.

Does that mean you don't have sex? Or you don't like it, or you don't need it, or you haven't done it?

It must mean all of that. I just don't think about sex. It's too dirty and disgusting. Don't you think so?

No—I like it. Are you happy about the way you feel?

Yes, I am happy.

Rossano Brazzi

Studio 54 is the link between Andy Warhol and Rossano Brazzi. "Andy" is synonymous with "Studio"—and that's where I met Rossano on his first visit. His wife was carrying their little white Pekinese, while the photographer captured the incongruity of a dog at Studio 54. We talked the following day in his suite at the Pierre, while his wife (to whom he has been married since he was twenty-one) sat in the next room. Rossano is likable, gallant, courteous, with the deeply romantic resonant voice and vibrant blue eyes which contributed to his image of stereotypical Latin lover, known to millions in films like *South Pacific*, *Summertime*, and *A Certain Smile*.

To me Rossano Brazzi is the Italian man personified, so I started by testing one of my theories about Italian men. Almost every woman who visits Italy is drenched by love poems and love declarations from ardent Latin lovers. I always imagined flattery to be the mainstay of the Italian male's seduction kit. So I asked Rossano Brazzi if he agreed with Richard Burton's advice to tell every woman she is beautiful. But Rossano caught me unaware by disagreeing and putting minimum emphasis on flowery compliments.

Like Barry Newman, Rossano Brazzi could be labeled macho. Like Rod Steiger, he stresses the importance of not confusing love with sex. And, startlingly, Rossano Brazzi is the first of my male interviewees to reveal that he lost his virginity when he was very, very young.

I was always known as the Latin lover. I've made 223 pictures and acted with 223 leading ladies. I remember working in Hollywood studios where men would say, "He is a great lover," or "She is a great lover." And I would laugh—because greatness in bed is a combination of two people. To give and to take is what makes a good lover.

I don't like lines or routines. Words *are* important in sex, but not all the time, not as a rule, not with every woman. I don't agree that you should tell every woman that she is beautiful. For example, I made *Summertime* with Katharine Hepburn—we were very good friends—but if I had said, "Kathy, you are beautiful," she would have laughed. Because she knows for herself that she is not beautiful—but she has got so many other things that at the right time she could become more than beautiful.

There are so many beautiful women—but sex doesn't always go with beauty. I made *Little Women* with Elizabeth Taylor when she was seventeen. She was beautiful, but I don't find her sexy. I imagine that she is—but she is not what *I* idealize as a sexy woman. I knew Marilyn Monroe very well—she was sexy, could create passion in a man, and was beautiful as well. Marilyn had a catlike quality—she was very soft, with beautiful skin, and her eyes were a great contrast to her body. She had something special within her that came out in her eyes. My ideal woman would have Marilyn's mouth and skin, Cyd Charisse's legs—or Mitzi Gaynor's now (I made *South Pacific* with her twenty years ago), Maria Felix's eyes, and something of Katharine Hepburn's character. Nothing of an Italian woman: not Sophia Loren. We made a picture together with John Wayne. We were in the desert together and Sophia and I had to share a bath. Sophia is too violent for me—too Neapolitan.

A man is stronger than a woman—he is the lion and the woman is the lamb. The man always feels he must control the woman—not because he is a dictator, but because he is the male. And a woman should wait and let the man approach her. A woman who makes advances is the most terrible thing. I blush if a woman approaches me. I lose my pride—I find it so aggressive. A woman should always be shrewd and show the man aspects of herself that will please him, then he will always approach her.

The man will recognize the right moment in which to approach a woman. If there is something between a man and a woman, then there will be a sort of electricity—the most important rapport between a man and a woman. Something which goes with sex, with feeling, with mind. Then a man will feel it and can be sure. A man has to feel it—to feel something for the woman: what a volcano, what warmth. At moments like that a man feels that he has really got a heart that is not just a muscle but that reacts to an emotion. But you have to feel the attraction in reality—then the approach will come naturally. It is the same as acting—if you really feel the role you don't have to think, "I must do this, I must look over there, I must do that." Because if you feel the role, then everything will come naturally. It is the same with a woman.

Physical love is the last part of a relationship for me. If I meet a girl at a party I am first interested in her mind and her conversation—*then* I notice that she has got beautiful eyes and a good smile. You can find a woman who appeals to you physically on a night when you are in a special mood—then for that night you can have a most beautiful relationship. I believe in going to bed in that way—but one must always remember that that is passion and not love.

I believe that women get more pleasure out of sex then men. After making love a woman's pleasure goes on and on, but a man's stops. It is also difficult to know when a woman has an orgasm and when she is faking. A man may not realize a woman is faking the first time she does it. But he ought to know the third or fourth time, if he has a rapport with her.

I made love for the first time when I was ten. I was ill in bed with a bad leg, and one Thursday my father and mother and the maid had to go out. So they asked the niece of a friend to look after me. Her name was Tosca—she was nineteen and she had already had an affair with her fiancé. She started to touch me and I made love to her. I knew exactly what to do and it was beautifully exciting, even though I wasn't fully developed. Later, my father found out and the girl was sent away. After that I didn't go out with a woman until I was sixteen. Then the physical rapport was very beautiful, but I knew I had to control myself like a man.

Looking back, having since been to medical school, I know that having sex so young can be bad for a boy. There was a nine-year-old boy who died because his nurse played with him—there was a big trial in Florence and she got twenty years in prison.

If I had to advise a man on how to be good in bed, I would tell him to make love for a long time. An American man I knew was married to a young Italian girl and they were having physical trouble because the man finished making love before he had hardly started. His wife was getting fed up, so I gave him some advice: "You mustn't go to bed, jump on your wife, make love—then stop. There are so many other things to do. First of all there is kissing." My friend said, "But of course I kiss my wife—and on the mouth." I said, "That is not enough—if you really love your wife you will want to eat her." And my friend said, "But Rossano, I vomit." So I said, "Well—you are married to a young Italian girl, and if you want to keep her . . ." When I went back to America a year later, the marriage was going really well and the husband told me that he hadn't realized what he had been missing. I think it is cruel for a man not to do that for a woman.

An Italian man never just jumps on his wife—he starts by eating her. My mother used to say, "Rossano, you were born from there and you will die there."

In America men have problems with women because they can't divide themselves between their work and love. They are too interested in work and money, money, money. In Italy we think love is more important. Italians are inclined to forget everything the moment they are with a woman. You see, we have a Neapolitan saying: "The thing of a man can't have worries, because if it has worries it won't work." A man has to forget everything while he is making love—even his wife, if he has got one—forget everything, and then he will be a good lover.

Giancarlo Gianinni

Swept Away star Giancarlo Gianinni is today's archetypal latin lover. He shares Rossano Brazzi's dislike of aggressive women, but modifies this by saying that liberated women are usually sweet in bed. Giancarlo also denigrates flattery, but admits that it still remains the tactic of some Italian men. And like Rossano, Giancarlo reveals that he lost his virginity before his teens.

Lina Wertmuller introduced me to Giancarlo Gianinni when they were both in New York to promote their first American film, *A Night Full of Rain*. I had hoped to interview Lina, but she said she didn't want to be the only director in the book, and asked me to interview a male director. But by the time I found one, Lina Wertmuller had already left for Italy. Nevertheless, I spoke to Giancarlo, in his suite at the Sherry-Netherland. I interviewed him in a bizarre mixture of Italian and French, and he answered in Italian, punctuated with a few tentative words of English. The interview sounds very romantic on tape, and in person, Giancarlo's soulful blue eyes equaled their on-screen impact.

I have no problems about sex. I only worried about sex once in my life. I was with a woman who was very aggressive—as aggressive as ten women put together. So I promised myself never to see her again. I don't like very aggressive women—I know a lot of liberated women and they are usually very sweet in bed. In *Swept Away* I played a man who is very dominant—but I have only slapped a woman once in my life. Five years ago I had a fight with my wife—not just about sex but about other things. I slapped her and she punched me back. Otherwise I have never hit a woman.

Italian men have the reputation of being such great lovers, but I don't know why. I do know that many Italians, especially the southern Italians, are used to flattering women. But I am not like that. Words are not so important to me in sex, because when I look into a woman's eyes I understand everything. A woman's eyes are most important to me. Of course one can also take a woman's hands and send or receive a message. One can also talk—but one needn't say, "Let's go to bed."

When things go wrong sexually I believe the mistake is always the man's—he is guilty, because he doesn't understand the woman. Every woman is different, and a man needs to be special with every woman and to make her realize that she is completely special. Every woman needs a different kind of loving. I have learned from being with many, many women that a type of woman doesn't exist. For me all women are the same the world over—because all women are different, and so are the same in being different.

A man has to change himself for every woman he is with, because just as every woman is different, so is every relationship. When I talk to a woman and look into her eyes I feel something, know I want to be with her, and am completely different than I was with another woman I was with the day before.

Sex is one of the most important things in life. I began when I was eleven in Sardinia. I was afraid because my friends had told me that it would be difficult—that nothing would happen. The girl was eighteen. I said, "This is the first time—please help me," and she did—she was very kind. So the sex was very sweet and wonderful. After that it was three years until I had another relationship with a woman. Then many, many other women—why not? It was like a school.

What is the secret of being good in bed? There isn't a method; you can't teach it. It's in my character. When I was little it was very difficult because I was very shy—maybe that's the reason I started having sex when I was eleven. I can explain it in terms of acting. I went on stage because I was shy, as a contrast. When an actor is shy he is generally a good actor once he is on stage; he changes, he does many things—that is what makes him a good actor. And the same qualities are what makes a man good in bed.

Helmut Berger

Helmut Berger is blond, charming, and witty and has been labeled "the most handsome man in the world." Star of many films, including Visconti's *The Damned*, Helmut Berger, like Rossano Brazzi and Giancarlo Giannini, lives in Rome. An immensely eligible bachelor, Helmut has been romantically linked to some of the world's most glamorous and notorious women. Unafraid of controversy, Helmut frankly admitted his own bisexuality long before such admissions became fashionable.

I phoned Helmut Berger in Rome, and we talked for an hour before he agreed to an interview. Polite, articulate, and intelligent, Helmut questioned me, tested me—finally pronounced, "You are not bitchy," and invited me to interview him in Rome. A date was set. Helmut also arranged for me to interview his friend Ursula Andress, but at the last minute circumstances forced me to cancel. I finally interviewed Helmut Berger at the Sherry-Netherland in New York, two hours before he was due to fly to Paris. In person, as on the telephone, Helmut was charming and courteous, but more masculine than I had expected. He talked to me openly, and his attitudes toward love, sex, and relationships strike a delicate balance between European romanticism and American permissiveness. In fact I think "delicate balance" is the phrase which best describes Helmut Berger: he manages to combine poise with abandon, elegance with informality, remoteness with warmth, jet-setting with professionalism, masculinity with sensitivity. And Helmut Berger is the only man I have ever met who, as a casual acquaintance, could call me "darling" and not sound phony.

I am against analyzing sex too much, because too much analysis creates lack of spontaneity. If I fall in love with a man and first analyze my feelings, then I don't do anything. If I fall in love with a woman and analyze too much, I become scared of certain attitudes, probably produced by women's lib.

Can you define the different attitudes to sex in Europe and America?

In America men are completely controlled by women. America is totally a woman's country. Europe

is still a man's country. I prefer that; I like women to
be very feminine, and I think that women's lib has
changed American women. I like women who still take
care of a man; I want a woman to be a wife, a mother,
a lover, and a child, and I love a woman to be intelligent. Americans take sex very seriously, but they also
rush too much. The scene in *Network* where Faye
Dunaway talks about work while she makes love mirrors the American way of loving. Everything is
business and money, money, money. Men think, "I
must be in the office at nine." They rush and rush till
they become impotent. They only make love on Satur-
day night. It is all too planned, too controlled, and I
am against it. The Germans also make love like the
Americans—they rush and they plan. But in Italy we
make love by moonlight, we take time, we don't fix a
time for sex. You have to make love when you feel it,
where you feel it. For me there is no fixed time or
place for sex. I had sex in a plane, had sex in different
places, at different times. I am very free.

How did you become sexually free?

Some of it is born. I never had any sexual complexes. I think it is because I love to give. I sometimes
feel that I am sexually perfect—because each person
I've been involved with has stayed and was wanted to
be with me after years. I was brought up as a
Catholic—by the Franciscans—and I was at college till
I was eighteen. Sex was very religious, and the woman
was treated like a Madonna. Once I got punished because they said I looked at a girl as if I were un-
dressing her with my eyes. After I left college it took
me five years to transcend the education I received
there. But eventually I had a very special relationship,
which acted like a green light and taught me to be sexually free. Now nothing shocks me about sex, except
incest and child prostitution—all sex is perfect for me.
But I do still find it difficult to pick someone up. I like
to flirt, but I can only flirt to a certain point; then I

withdraw. Each time I flirt with someone I do want to go to bed with them, but before it happens I am very nervous. People are frightened when they meet me, before we go to bed—so I have to play myself down. People today are scared of showing their feelings, of losing control.

How would you describe flirting?

Paying attention to a woman. You have to circle a woman like an animal does. You have to build up a relationship with words, gifts, attentions. You have to build up the woman by making her feel fantastic, that she is super-beautiful, the best in town. It is very important to give a woman confidence—a woman needs to relax and feel secure. You have to build up her confidence, build up the relationship—sex is only the second step, to be taken once the flirting stage is over.

How do you discover what someone wants sexually?

First of all you have to get under the covers—and once you are under the covers you get a feeling about the other person. It also depends on their intelligence and sensitivity. Some people are less sensitive, others more. If someone is not sensitive then you have to talk about the sex.

How important to you are sex fantasies?

One has a lot of fantasy during masturbation—but I don't have more pleasure in masturbating than I do when I make love to someone. You have sex fantasies during masturbation, but you also incorporate those fantasies into the sex you have with someone else. You create. I like creating a relationship, building something with someone—doing things with them. And I am faithful if I love someone.

Do you feel love and sex should be related?

The best sex is always with the person you love—otherwise it is only sex. Without love sex is just jerking off. But it is always a problem finding the right person to love. You have to wait if you really want strong, sincere love. I've had the best—but now I wait. I won't give myself for minor experiences—why should I? So I wait. I know exactly that one day I am going to meet the right person. Man or woman—I don't mind as long as they are the right person and I love and am loved.

What is the difference between being a good lover for a woman and being a good lover for a man?

I don't think there is any difference. It is no more difficult to bring a man to an orgasm than it is with a woman—it *is* easy for a man to get a hard-on, but difficult for him to come in the right way. Sometimes one orgasm can be better than ten—and other times ten orgasms can seem like one. The important thing in a relationship with a man or a woman is for both of you to educate one another sexually. To know what you like, to discover what the other person likes, being open sexually, creating a sexual experience in the form of a rainbow. You have to love—but with patience and understanding. You have to try to be sexually free. The bedroom isn't Trafalgar Square, or Fifth Avenue, it is your room, your life. The bedroom is your life. And you must remember that you can only learn to be sexually free through an important relationship; you can't learn to be sexually free with hookers, you can only learn to be sexually free with someone you love.

Prince Egon Von Furstenberg

Austrian, like Helmut Berger, Prince Egon Von Furstenberg reminds me of a refugee from a Viennese operetta, one of Stauss' or Romberg's blond, blue-eyed, handsome heros. Until he smiles—then the gap in his teeth and the glint in his eyes hint at a strain of appealing wickedness. Thirty-three years old, a noted designer of men's wear, creator of his own fragrance, and author of *The Power Look,* Egon is related to two of Europe's most prestigious families, the Von Furstenbergs and the Agnellis; his uncle Gianni Agnelli is Fiat czar and one of the most powerful men in the world. Egon is separated from his beautiful designer wife, Diane, but they are still the best of friends. Both are highly visible in international society.

In effect, I hijacked Egon Von Furstenberg for this interview. After I arrived at Diane's house to interview her, I found the interview had been postponed, and met Egon, in the process of visiting his two children. I described my book and he agreed to an interview, and we left for his apartment and immediately started the interview. Egon was forthcoming, laughed a lot, was definite, pausing only fractionally after each question before answering frankly in his Austrian accent. Prince Egon Von Furstenberg's frankness may surprise some people—and in the past he and Diane have shocked New York society with intimate revelations about their sex lives. Here, Egon talks with characteristic openness about losing his virginity at thirteen, and experiencing sex in strange places. Prince Egon Von Furstenberg's views on women and sex are liberated and in harmony with the sexual revolution.

Do you think a man is born good in bed?

I think a man is definitely born with more or less of a tendency for sex. The first time I ever made love to a woman, I was thirteen and she was a German hooker. She was very nice—I made love to her three times that night and I really liked it.

What advice will you give your son and daughter about sex?

I will tell my son to start very early. I will tell my daughter to choose a man she respects. I don't think I will advise anything else—it depends on her. But I think she *will* start early. My sister got married at fifteen—she was very grown-up.

How would you describe the best way to approach a woman?

You can tell if a woman is interested in you by looking into her eyes and by shaking her hand. Then you have to study the woman and discover her weak and her strong points. You have to look at the way she moves, how she talks to other people, watch how she bites her nails and how she moves her hair. Then you have to try to say something that appeals to the woman. So that if you are with an insecure woman, you try to make her feel secure. If you are with a secure woman you have to play baby, tell her your problems so that she feels she has to protect you. A man has to catch a woman with his brains and not his looks.

Richard Burton says you should tell every woman that she is beautiful. Do you agree?

I think women appreciate that. But you can't tell every woman that she is beautiful. You have to tell some women that they move well, or that they really turn you on.

Do you think the man should always initiate the relationship?

No. I think a woman should be honest and tell a man he is great and that she fancies him—if she really does. If a woman knows how to flatter a man, she has him right away—because men don't get flattered enough. If a woman really wants to approach a man, then she should. I once met a girl at a disco—we weren't properly introduced and just said hello. She smiled at me, then the next day phoned me. She asked if I remembered her, I said no, whereupon she said, "I would like to have dinner with you." I said okay—went to meet her—and we stayed together for a year. Sex can be very chemical between two people—either it works well, or it doesn't.

How do you think a man should communicate what he wants sexually?

I think he can show the woman, without asking for it. I also think a man should discover what the woman wants with her help—by her showing him. Two people need to get to know each other. Then they can talk about sex—not on the first or second night, but later on. At that point it is easier to talk about sex. I also think it is very nice to speak during sex.

What kind of advice would you give to men who want to discover what kind of woman they are with?

Sweet women are usually very sensitive and very strong; outgoing women usually want to be really put-down in sex. I am basically a not very complicated person—I don't believe in tying someone to the wall—but I am definitely more on the sadistic than the masochistic side, so sadistic women don't last long with me.

How important is the woman's orgasm to you?

In America the orgasm is talked about such a lot. That is very depressing—very cold. I don't think a man should ask if a woman has come. Sometimes you don't really know if the woman has come the first time you are with her. But an American woman will usually tell you and say something like "I didn't—let's start again." European women don't tell you if they haven't had an orgasm, but still make the effort to see you again. I think, though, that women do become more affectionate if they have had an orgasm. I have also been told that you can tell if a woman has had an orgasm because her bosom becomes very soft. Also, it turns me on if I make love to a woman while she masturbates. She knows herself best, so I can learn how to please her—because she does it better than I would—and it really turns me on.

What makes a man bad in bed?

Unresponsiveness. And the major problem is obviously being unable to—because then there is no sex. The man can give the woman head, but . . . Although I do enjoy giving head to a woman; I've always enjoyed it. But not many women know how to suck a man's cock well. They should take in as much as possible and try not to bite. But more and more women are improving.

What do you think women really want sexually from men?

Women want a man next to them to whom they can really relate. Then they want a man who pleases them. They want a man who gives them good sex. Women are pleased by having good sex—by coming at the same time as the man they are with. I think that you build up to good sex with the relationship, and by talking. Situations can also make sex very good—if you have sex in a strange place where you would never think of having sex, like on a staircase. A woman once gave me head on a plane in the loo—I was petrified and came after two seconds.

What advice would you give to men who want to be good in bed?

I think you have to be very free in sex and remember that nothing is vulgar—everything is allowed if it gives you pleasure. You have to know when to be soft and when to be hard, to recognize the feeling of the moment. You can tell by how a woman starts to build up—it's instinctive. You have to be really sweet sometimes—but not always.

I think it's terrible if one goes to bed with a man for sex and he pretends to be romantic and loving when really there is no love involved. How important do you think love is to sex?

Not very. But if I knew I were going to die tomorrow and could only have one more sexual experience I would choose to sleep with someone I love very much—and to cuddle them.

Peter Frampton

Peter Frampton is not one to tell tales of groupie sex. It's not his style. Instead the British-born rock superstar revealed how he lost his virginity in an alleyway, the times he didn't enjoy sex, how sleeping around turns him off, and how, with Barry Newman, Egon Von Furstenberg, and Rossano Brazzi, he also has had difficulty in recognizing the female orgasm. Throughout the interview Peter referred to his then girlfriend Penny McCall, who later sued him for alimony.

I met Peter Frampton's manager on the set of *Sergeant Pepper's Lonely Heart's Club Band,* at MGM in Hollywood. Frampton's manager was in the process of refusing my request for an interview with his client when Peter Frampton came over to me, smiled, and said, "I saw you on TV being interviewed about your book on women—I thought it sounded great." Predictably, I said, "Thank you. Would you like to be in the next one?" Peter Frampton said yes—and later that week, we met in his trailer at MGM. Peter was dressed in black satin and wore mirror-lens glasses, which he removed when we began to talk. He was shy, tentative, but relaxed as the interview progressed. After the interview, I chatted to Peter's parents, who were visiting L.A.—a nice middle-class English couple, enjoying their son's phenomenal success. Twenty-eight-year-old Peter Frampton is shy, sensitive, and gentle—a rock superstar of the '70s.

I always thought I was terrible in bed. I was about fifteen when I first had sex—in an alley outside a gig I was playing. I didn't know what I was supposed to do. I can't remember all the details—I don't even know whether we did it properly. I hope I've changed a lot sexually since then—before Penny there were times when I didn't enjoy sex at all. It wasn't really making love, it was just finding it then wondering what the hell to do next.

I was very shy and I never used to be able to talk a girl into going to bed with me in the first place. I'd walk up to a girl, then freeze—my mouth didn't work at all and I was speechless. I didn't have very much confidence in myself in even just talking—forget about sex. You just get passed over by women if you don't have personality.

At this point, women are coming on to me very strongly because of my career. I've never been the sort of person who has stuck out—or has even wanted to. But now I get confronted by people who think I've got to be somebody special—which I'm not. But in a way I've asked for it and I've got to deal with it. Penny really helped me—she showed me how to look at myself and believe in myself. She gave me a lot of confidence that I was a nice person.

I've always been a basically monogamous person, even though men are meant to be polygamous. I'm not saying I've never been with a groupie—but sleeping around really turns me off completely. Unfortunately my first marriage didn't work out, so when it started to go bad, I started sleeping around, but I didn't enjoy it. I wasn't really looking for a new chick every night—I was looking for a long-term relationship. I think sex is very important in a relationship—but equally that the two heads are on the same wavelength. For me, good sex was being with the right lady. Penny was the first woman in my life to make me feel like I was a superman in bed. Sex is very much an ego thing, and there's nothing better than someone turning around and saying, "You are fantastic in bed." I think I've been with some women in my life who haven't enjoyed sex. When I first started having sex I couldn't tell if the woman had really climaxed, but now it is really important to me if the woman climaxes when I make love to her.

I suppose the man has to be the leader in sex, but it's nice when the woman takes over to be able to switch off. I don't think a man should tell a woman what he wants—especially not at first. But one can experiment later on, which is a lot of fun. Sex is like an adventure—you try a lot of things, then if you get a good reaction you have discovered what the woman wants. Sex would be very boring for me if I talked about it and planned it out, because I ad-lib all the time—in my music and in my lovemaking.

Anson Williams

I wanted to label Anson Williams's interview "All-American Boy"—but although that was apt, I decided "Happy Days" would be more appropriate—a reminder of his role as Potsie in the hit TV series. Zsa Zsa Gabor introduced me to Anson while they were both taping a Hollywood game show. Zsa Zsa remarked on Anson's handsome, clean-cut looks, the sort every mother would welcome in a son-in-law. After the show we all had dinner at the studio. Then I interviewed Anson in his dressing room, while Buddy Hackett, also in the show, sat in a corner, silently presiding over us. A rising singing and acting star, aware of the sharks lurking under Hollywood's glittery surface, Anson warned me about being cheated in business. Sharp, but managed protectively by his father, Anson Williams still retains an all-American innocence.

Anson Williams and Peter Frampton, in the same age group, share similar attitudes; they both dislike one-night-stands and women who are too aggressive, and both place primary importance on love and caring.

I think young people today are going back to really caring. To thinking and deciding about relationships instead of just jumping into bed. I don't think we are more permissive than people were fifty years ago—sex is just out in the open now, instead of behind closed doors. But there are still people around who overintellectualize mates and sex. They try to find reasons for everything instead of just doing it. I think people should stop defining their feelings and go more with "I like this person."

I think you have to be a best friend to a woman before you can be her best lover. To know her better than you know yourself. A good lover takes the time to find out about the woman beforehand—he is honest, has the desire to please her, cares about her, considers her, and is unselfish. I don't think any good affairs happen by jumping into the sack immediately—you really have to care for and treasure the woman you are with.

I have always been a feminist—I think women are wonderful, terrific, and that God gave them ingredients that men don't possess; a magic and an intuitiveness. Women are equal to men and have the same desires and needs as I do. But I think women get more pleasure out of sex than men do, judging by the women I have known. Women are designed to have more pleasure in sex, but then again, they also have more pain in childbirth.

There are women who are too aggressive, and I don't like that. Women who come on too strong and go beyond the boundaries into my territory. I don't like pushy people. Especially when I am in a concert I meet women who just ask me to go to bed with them—they are pretty blunt. But I won't go to bed with women like that because they are trying to use me—I'd be a fool to go with them because they make me feel like a prostitute.

Any affairs I've had have been fifty-fifty, very mutual. I don't think I have ever gone up to a girl and said, "Do you want to go to bed?" It is very chauvinistic to think a man should ask. Sex is a mutual thing; when it is right to go to bed, then it is right. I don't believe in lines or games, or trying to use somebody. I am as honest as I can possibly be. I try to take as much pride in what I am and in my being. I try to do what I do on this earth as best I can—and when it comes to making love I do what I do best. Everyone has his own way of making love, but I think that should be private. Everything depends on the mate you are with. There is no one person who is the world's greatest lover—it's all individual.

A good lover doesn't always have to be ready to make love. I believe in quality, not quantity. I don't think you should try to be a good lover—but instead try to be a good man. Because I don't believe you become a better lover by copying someone's techniques; you become a better lover by having a loving heart.

In Part I, "The Experts," Tish Baldrige, Erika Padan Freeman, and Emerson Symonds point to a new trend among young people which Anson Williams characterizes: "I think young people today are going back to really caring, to thinking and deciding about relationships, instead of just jumping into bed." And the male celebrities do express changes in attitudes to love, sex, and relationships. I have summarized the male celebrities' sexual attitudes, and their advice to other men.

SUMMARY OF SEXUAL ATTITUDES

1. Good in bed is endowment.
2. Good in bed is being able to come three or four times a night.
3. Good in bed is vitality.
4. The man should talk the woman into bed.
5. It doesn't matter who initiates sex.
6. The pleasure men and women get from sex is quite different.
7. Fantasies are very important.
8. You are either born with sexual imagination or not.
9. One night is too short a time to get to know the body of a woman.
10. A man should love, or *think* he loves, the woman.
11. Experience creates sexual confidence.
12. Some men know naturally how to touch.
13. If a man asks a woman to go to bed with him directly she will always say no.
14. The man is the dominant force.
15. A lot of men feel pressured into making love to a woman.
16. If the woman is too passive, then the man finds it hard to get mentally stimulated.
17. If the woman is too aggressive, then it's hard for the man to get emotionally stimulated.
18. It's easier for women than for men to have sex.
19. If a man feels pressured to make a woman orgasm, then he won't enjoy the sex.

20. Guys go through a certain stage in life when they have a lot of sex, but deep down they would prefer to have a woman to make them happy that they make happy.

21. Sex with the woman you love has got to be the best sex.

22. Stamina and staying power have nothing to do with being good in bed.

23. To give and to take makes a good lover.

24. Words are important—but not with every woman.

25. A man always feels he must control the woman. ?

26. It is difficult to know when a woman has an orgasm and when she is faking.

27. If the sex goes wrong it is always the man's fault.

28. You can't teach being good in bed.

29. Sleeping around is a complete turnoff.

30. Sex is very much an ego thing—and there is nothing better than the woman turning around and saying, "You are fantastic in bed."

31. It is really important to a man if a woman climaxes.

32. Men masturbate more than women, so they want something extra—warmth and tenderness—when they go to bed with a woman.

33. A man shouldn't try to be a good lover.

SUMMARY OF SEXUAL ADVICE

1. Make love for a long time.
2. Give a woman oral sex.
3. Forget everything while you are making love.
4. Change with every woman.
5. Study a woman and discover her strong and weak points. Watch the way she moves and talks to other people.
6. If you are with an insecure woman, try to make her feel secure.
7. If you are with a secure woman, play baby—tell

her your problems so she feels she has to protect you.

8. Catch a woman with brains, not looks.

9. Tell a woman that she is beautiful, or that she turns you on.

10. Talk about sex—but not on the first or second night.

11. Have sex in strange places.

12. Try to recognize the feeling of the moment.

13. Be very free in sex and remember that nothing is vulgar.

14. Try a lot of things—then if you get a good reaction you have discovered what the woman wants.

15. Never ask a woman to go to bed with you verbally.

16. Judge if a woman wants to go to bed with you by her eyes—you can see her pupils enlarging if she is attracted to you.

17. If you want to do something sexually, start doing it.

18. Don't suppress the feminine part of your makeup.

19. Clichés are the best approach to a woman.

20. Make a woman feel comfortable.

21. Be very slow and warm the woman up to a point of no return.

22. Talk to a woman in bed.

23. Talk about sex after bed—not before.

24. Don't worry about sex or feel it has to be perfect each time.

25. Learn all about a woman's body.

26. Be open and honest.

In the next section, the female celebrities criticize some of the sexual attitudes expressed by the male celebrities in this section. They also corroborate and contradict, quarrel with and approve of some of the sexual advice male celebrities gave in this section.

Part III

The
Female Celebrities

The male celebrities talked about their sexual fears; here female celebrities tell if those fears are justified. The male celebrities talked about liberated women: here liberated women talk about men. The male celebrities talked about their desires; here the female celebrities reveal how those desires match or conflict with their own. In the last section, male celebrities talked about what they try to be; in this section female celebrities talk about what they want to experience—what they want from men in bed.

The interviews are set out as in the last section, roughly according to age group, and sometimes according to profession.

Topics Discussed

Apart from expressing their criticism of men, their sexual desires, and their advice to men, the female celebrities also tell how they feel about macho men, how they lost their virginity, how sex has changed in America since their teens, male sexual approaches, male sexual mistakes, male attitudes to the female orgasm, and the relationship between love and sex. The questions I asked will demonstrate other areas of discussion.

Questions to Interviewees

I asked female celebrities questions related to their image and their sexual preferences and desires. Many questions arose from my own experiences with men, others developed out of the conversation, and some subjects were discussed after a female celebrity had reacted negatively or positively to a male interview I showed her. These are the questions I asked:

What did your parents tell you about sex?

What did you hear about sex at school?

How did you feel when you lost your virginity?

Did that first sexual experience live up to your expectations?

How have you changed sexually since you lost your virginity?

How has the world changed for women since you grew up?

How do you think the women's liberation movement has affected relationships between men and women?

What kind of man do you think can cope with a liberated woman?

Do you think sex is more important to men than it is to women?

Do you think men care if women want them just for sex?

Do you care if a man wants you because of your image?

Do you really like sex?

Do you always want to have sex?

Are you ever disappointed with sex?

Have you ever wanted a man for just physical reasons?

Could you have sex with a stranger?

Could you have sex with a man you didn't love?

Could you have sex with a man who didn't love you?

Do you like a man to give you a lot of compliments?

What kind of pre-bed approach do you like?

Do you like it if a man tries to find out what you want sexually *before* bed?

How do you think a man should discover your fantasies and desires?

Do you think a man should ask for what he wants sexually?

Would you ever ask for what you wanted sexually?

Do you like it if a man asks if you have orgasmed?

Does it matter to you if you don't always have an orgasm?

Is it important to you if a man is good or bad in bed?

What do you think makes a man bad in bed?

What do you think makes a man good in bed?

Is it age?

Is it stamina?

Is it size?

Is it physical type?

Is it nationality?

Is it experience?

If you could create the ideal lover, what would he be like? Can you recognize the man who will be good for you *before* bed?

What advice would you give to a man who wants to be good in bed for you?

What, for you, makes good sex?

These questions are also the questions that I always want the man in my life to ask me, so that I can communicate my feelings about love, sex, and our relationship. My answers and the answers of the female celebrities—of any woman—reveal what women really want from men, what they feel about men, and exactly how women talk about men when men aren't around to listen.

Barbara Cartland

Barbara Cartland, the world's most popular romantic novelist, invited me to interview her at her
baronial home in Hertfordshire, England. Aware
that I was about to encounter a rare exponent of
virginity, I wore pale pink and lace, in an attempt
to appear as virginal as possible. Apparently to no
avail, because Mrs. Cartland was very icy. She
launched into a monologue; I tried to cut in, but
she clearly considered the subject demolished. Tea
was served, we chatted distantly, and I felt
uncomfortable, as if the pale pink of my dress had
deepened into telltale scarlet. Then, suddenly, in
the middle of the conversation, Mrs. Cartland
melted toward me. I don't know what secret but-
ton I accidentally pressed, but it was as if a sheet
of ice had slid from her face. Barbara became
warm and human, gave me advice about publish-
ers and contracts and introductions to seven of
her friends, and was genuinely kind to me. A few
weeks later, Barbara invited me to a private lunch
party. Afterward we strolled in her English country garden, talking about the Duchess of Windsor,
Lord Mountbatten of Burma, and an old world of
exclusivity and propriety.

Born near the turn of the century, Barbara
Cartland reflects on how fashions in manners, sex,
and relationships have altered since the First
World War, how women attained liberation, and
the price she believes men pay for that liberation.
At the same time, Barbara's sexual advice to men
is basic, and she illustrates what makes a man a
good lover with stories about legendary lovers. I
started this section with Barbara Cartland's inter-

view because I believe that her strong bias toward virginity, marriage, romance, and morality provides a base with which to compare the other female interviews that follow.

Love is part of the divine, something so special, so wonderful, so perfect, that one believes in the old legend, which says that the gods originally made one human being so perfect in every detail that the gods themselves became jealous. So they cut this creation in two, called it man and woman, and said that for the rest of their lives man and woman should always be seeking the other half of themselves. Only then would they find real happiness.

I think that that legend is so beautiful that every man and woman should remember it as a standard of what they want in life and in a partner.

Have attitudes to sex changed a great deal since you were growing up?

Men today are under great stress, eat the wrong food, and don't take enough exercise—with the result that they are not so sexually inclined as they were in previous generations. When the great Duke of Marlborough returned home from one of his conquests, he made love to his wife, Sarah, twice before even taking off his boots.

When I was young we were all very innocent. A young girl didn't have to fight for her virtue because nobody attacked it. There was an enormous gap between the lady and the prostitute. Men would take a girl like myself dancing and would never think of suggesting anything improper. They took a girl out because they admired her. They fell in love with her and wanted to marry her. After the First World War every man's idea of bliss was to come home, settle down with a wife, and have a family.

That was spoiled later on because men didn't have

the money to get married. In the meantime, girls got more promiscuous simply because contraception was easy and they weren't likely to have a baby every time they were touched. But in 1926 a doctor lecturing at Oxford University told the undergraduates that no woman was capable of feeling passion. Today we know women are just as capable of feeling passion as men.

But it's absolute rubbish—medically and from any other point of view—to talk about a man and a woman being equal when it comes to sex. They are certainly not equal. A man can have an "affair" which can mean absolutely nothing to him. He need never think of it again. It's the same as having a good meal; it's an entirely physical reaction. But that never, never happens with a woman because to them "making love" is always an emotional experience.

Don't you think women's liberation has had any effect?

Yes. Today's modern liberated women frighten men by confronting them with sex manuals and preconceived ideas of what should happen in bed—complaining, "I am entitled to this," or "Why aren't we doing that?" Many men are so frightened that they are either impotent or avoid women altogether. Other men feel that they have to indulge in all sorts of peculiar things they don't want to do and are terrified they will fail the false unnatural standards set by sex magazines. Men dislike women who want to compete and be liberated—men still feel chivalrous and romantic toward women.

If men want chivalry and romance, what do you think women want?

Women are still happiest when men are dominant. A woman wants to admire a man, to look up to him and respect him—so a man should be strong, resolute, determined, and masterful. I've never yet met a woman who wasn't happiest when her man was strong and possessive.

But women are also idealistic in love and still believe in a knight in shining armor ready to dedicate his life to them. So women need romance—every woman wants to know that she is important, that she is wanted and desired.

Before I was married I went dancing till dawn with a young man, and the next day some flowers arrived with a note: "Darling—I want these flowers to see you." I think that is wonderful wooing. Women want men who take them flowers and tell them over and over of their love.

It always annoys me when I ask a man if he loves me and he says, "You know I do." How do I know? I am not clairvoyant—a man has to tell me. I always taught my sons to remember birthdays and send flowers. It's up to a mother to bring up her sons to be romantic, because romance is what women want from men.

If you could create the ideal lover, what would he look like?

I create the ideal lover every day in my books—my heroes are always tall, dark, handsome, and cynical. The trouble is that I always thought I would be in love with men like that—but my men were usually blond, blue-eyed, and rather stupid.

Every woman's ideal lover looks like an ancient Greek athlete—or Michelangelo's *David.* Always tall—an ideal lover is never "short, dark, handsome"; violins never thrilled for Mickey Rooney and false eyelashes never fluttered for Edward G. Robinson.

The actors women admire on the screen are strong characters, tall men usually playing aggressive, often brutal roles—Richard Burton, Gregory Peck, Michael Caine.

What do you think makes a man a good lover?

Part of it—the physical, not the spiritual—is self-control. A good lover has the power of self-control. The late Prince Aly Khan, who was reputedly the greatest lover of the '30s and '40s, was taught the process of *imsak* by an Egyptian. In Arabian *imsak* means "holding" or "retaining." Prince Aly was supposed at one time to have had three mistresses simultaneously on three different floors of the Ritz Hotel. And he satisfied them all each night—but he himself only reached climax twice a week.

Obviously the average man won't be like that, but any man should excite a woman with his hands, his words, and his lips for as long as possible before ending his lovemaking.

So much in sex depends on the man; I think it is his fault if the woman doesn't respond. But there is no need for a wife to know anything more than what her husband is prepared to teach her.

You say the man has to teach the woman to make love. Doesn't the woman have any influence on the man's lovemaking?

I think a man has to be flattered into believing he is a good lover long before he is, and after a man has made love to a woman she ought to tell him he was wonderful. The more a woman tells a man he is wonderful, the more wonderful he becomes.

Men often fail sexually because they are frightened of being rejected. A woman has to be understanding and tactful and must always realize that failure can happen. So many different things can put a man off sex and upset the impetus of his desire—a noise in the bedroom next door, his wife using the wrong scent.

Also when men get older they worry about the infrequency of their desire, and worrying makes it worse. They need to be reminded that there is no age limit on sexual arousal—the late Marquess of Donegall was conceived when his father was over ninety.

What advice would you give a man who wanted to be good in bed?

Don't rush at a woman like a bull—that will shock her. Lovemaking should really be the end of a long, long kiss. And if a man loves a woman he won't do anything to shock her. The important thing is to take the trouble to find the woman's erogenous zones and to realize that while kissing one woman on her neck may excite her to madness, the same thing may fail to excite any response in another woman.

Out of the billions and billions of bodies in the world it is the greatest miracle of creation that no one is exactly the same as another.

But if a man is healthy, if he avoids tension, takes the right amount of exercise, eats pure foods and plenty of protein, everything will work out properly.

Concentration is very important. Men should remember that the act of love is far more important than the contract he is drawing up for a new product. It is far more important than the board meeting he is going to attend tomorrow.

I say, then, give your full attention to love and sex at least for that moment. Make it not only physical, but something beautiful and divine—which it should be.

However successful you may become, if you do not have the happiness of loving and being loved, you are a failure as a man. Love, both physical and spiritual, makes a man what he should be—a supreme creation in the image of God.

Phyllis Diller

I interviewed Phyllis Diller in her suite at the Savoy Hotel, London, on my birthday. She offered me champagne to celebrate, and we talked for half an hour. Phyllis had little pink plastic roses in her hair (like the kind used for birthday-cake candle holders) and wore a blue chiffon caftan and diamonds. The diamonds were nevertheless eclipsed by Phyllis Diller's beautiful topaz eyes, which obviously no one can attribute to plastic surgery or beauty parlors. Phyllis was warm and friendly, sometimes redirecting the questions back to me—so when I asked her about male approaches, Phyllis said, "Men don't approach me. But you are a different type—you are a very beautiful fluffball—so you will be approached by all types of men." I am not sure if that was a compliment, but I do know that Phyllis Diller was a very open, likable, direct, and professional interviewee.

Phyllis Diller and Barbara Cartland belong to the same generation. Although Phyllis's language is decidedly more basic than Barbara's, she too longs for romance and denigrates women's liberation. Yet Phyllis still sounds liberated, believing that a woman should teach a man to please her, and emphasizes the importance of her orgasm. Phyllis Diller's interview is racy, blunt, thoughtful, and very specific, especially on the subject of male endowment.

I work with audiences every night and I find people are people. Everybody laughs at the same things, everybody is hurt by the same things, therefore everybody is alike—and there is only good sex and bad sex.

What do you think makes a man good?

The ideal man is sensitive and cares about how the other person feels. Really, men should stop being so uptight about being good lovers and just do what comes naturally. But if a man is worrying about sex and making love he should listen to instruction from a female. It's often unfortunate being the woman to teach a young man—because experienced men are much better than beginners; they have been taught by many women.

How would you teach a beginner?

While he is making love you tell him what he is doing right and what he is doing wrong. You teach him while you are doing it. And the next thing you know you'll have an expert. Although a man can reach ninety and still won't have learned anything because he is a bad sex partner.

If I could teach a man I'd try to teach him to change—not always do the same thing, or want the same thing, to play moods and fantasies.

I don't agree. When I go to bed I'm me. And I don't mind sex becoming a habit—because if it's good habitually then that's wonderful.

Do you think a man should ask for what he wants sexually?

I think there should be a mutual telling. It's very simple; all those old jokes—there are certain places where one is physically sensitive, and if a person isn't hitting a certain spot I think it's perfectly correct to say "higher" or "lower."

What kind of an initial approach do you like from a man before bed?

Men don't approach me—I'm not an approachable woman and I never have been; I wasn't even an approachable child. I was bright, and boys don't approach bright girls. They are a threat, so that being bright and funny was a double threat, because boys were afraid they might be made fun of or made the butt of a joke. The male ego is the most delicate thing in the world. It is nurtured in such a way that it is supposed to be solid rock—and isn't allowed to be human. So men assume the role of being completely impervious to any ego threats. That's why you get men who go to singles bars wanting sex but no marriage or responsibility. Men like that are out for conquest. I am old-fashioned—I don't believe in a guy coming up to you in the street and saying, "Hey, babe—let's go to bed." There are American films where people meet, rent a hotel room, go to bed, make love all day, then discover each other's name six hours later. I'm not into that.

Could you have sex with someone you didn't love?

No—I don't think so. I think a good lover always tells you he loves you when he comes—and that can't happen if you are jumping on a different person every night, because then it would be a lie.

What attracts you to a man?

I'm a sucker for beauty—be it in a man, a woman, a child, a house, or a car. Both my husbands were very attractive. If there is ever a choice in anything I'll always choose beauty—even if it means giving up other qualities that are equally necessary. The thing that gets me is an attractive man who treats me like a lady. I'm a candlelight-and-romance lady—and I can't compromise in anything because I know that you can get romance if you wait long enough for that man to come along. It starts with conversation, then kissing, then both of you beginning to feel the same way—that's romance.

Do you think women's liberation has changed things?

No. It will always be the same, and women's liberation is never going to change relationships between men and women. I don't go along with women's lib. I don't really like it. I'm a third-generation career girl, so I've always been liberated and I take it for granted. And I like being a woman. Sex can be a great burden for men, though—because their role is still more important than women's. Men still have to act while all women have to do is react.

Does it matter to you to have an orgasm?

I think it's very important. There are all those jokes about wham, bang, thank you ma'am, and that's all wrong. You might as well be a pigeon. Sex should feel good from beginning to end. If you don't have an orgasm it might color your thinking about whether the man really cares about you. Ideally two people should come together—that's ideal.

How rare is the good-in-bed man?

I'd say one out of fifty.

Do you think stamina is important in a man?

It doesn't have anything to do with good sex.

What about size? I interviewed John Holmes, who is thirteen inches.

I consider that a freak. I'd just as soon go out with a dwarf. I think you ought to put an arrow on the end of it and say, "This is my knee." It's impossible if you have a man who is very largely endowed and a lady who is very small. I've had six children and I've still run up against something I couldn't handle (which certainly wasn't even thirteen inches). It's important that it matches. The key must fit the keyhole.

So it doesn't help?

My first husband had the greatest equipment in the world. He was a handsome man—beautifully endowed—but he refused to listen, to do an absolutely fine sex act. He would not do what felt good—all kinds of sex—oral anything. Wouldn't listen—wouldn't take any instruction. So he was a lousy sex partner, even though he had the greatest equipment and could have had great sex.

If you could create the ideal lover, what would he be like?

He would be my second husband—only sober. He was the perfect lover, because he was the perfect artistic lover, and for him sex was really an art form.

Regine

Regine is in agreement with Barbara Cartland that marriage is all. Her interview is the shortest in my book, but took longest to arrange. The trail to nightclub queen and social arbiter Regine began in March 1976, in Manhattan, where I met Regine's public-relations executive. She inspected the manuscript of my first book, and fortunately deemed that my project was fit for Regine. An interview was arranged, then disarranged. I spent the next six months missing Regine, who seemed forever frantically poised between Paris, Monte Carlo, Rio, and New York. Then, in Paris, in October 1976, I finally found the perfect entré— Prince Jean Poniatowski personally introduced me to Regine, and I even topped that by repeatedly meeting Regine at her Paris club. I felt that my credentials were cast-iron and that the interview was imminent. In New York in March 1977, yet another interview was arranged, then disarranged. Finally, in October 1977 in Beverly Hills, California, I phoned Regine at the Beverly Hills Hotel. I was informed that Regine was, not surprisingly, very busy, but I might possibly, just briefly, be seen, while Regine was in the midst of her manicure.

So at last, after nineteen months, Regine, in her bungalow at the Beverly Hills Hotel, being manicured. Surrounded by her entourage, attractive, without makeup, red hair matching mine. Surveying the scene, I remembered stories of kings and queens who held audiences for their subjects while they were eating, or being bathed. I talked to Regine for just fifteen minutes, during which time she hardly looked at me, or interrupted her manicure. I was sorry not to have more time with Regine, not because the wait merited it, but because I respect the saga of her self-made success and wanted to really meet the woman who had struggled, survived, and created an empire.

My period of sexual freedom was at a time when one talked about sex less—and had it more. My sole experience for years is my husband—and that continues to be a good experience—but we don't talk about sex, we do it. Even today when I go to bed with my husband I don't know in advance if we're going to make love—it just happens, and mostly we do. I am very cool—I am not obsessed with sex—because I don't have any sexual problems and I never have had. Today people talk about sex more—and do it less. The man will be good in bed if he excites the woman. A man can be terrible for ten women and wonderful for the eleventh. I don't truly think that you can tell if someone is going to be good in bed before you go to bed with them. Sex is a big mystery, and that is how it should be.

Frenchmen are very dedicated to lovemaking, but I don't think there's any nationality of men most likely to be good in bed. For me the most important thing is *une question de peau*—of skin—and of emotion. Of touch. You can touch someone, and suddenly it becomes the biggest affair in the world—there's a current, a chemistry, *une question de peau*. So that you both become part of the entire experience.

I was born liberated. Frankly I think that all women want to be married, that all women want to be with someone. And anything else they say they want is untrue. All women are bourgeois—they all want a home, they all want normality. And I believe that all women want a good husband—even if he isn't good in bed.

Monique Van Vooren

Belgian-born ex-Warhol star Monique Van Vooren is indelibly a part of Regine's glittering world. She is currently writing a novel, to be titled *Night Sanctuary*. Monique invited me to see her show at the Rainbow Grill, where she sang in a style reminiscent of Dietrich, but with a presentation all her own. We arranged to meet the next day at her elegant book-lined East Side apartment.

Monique was very honest, intelligent, and communicative, and I enjoyed talking to her. She went beyond what makes a man good in bed, specifying who is, was, or might be. Like Phyllis Diller, she doesn't rate stamina, and expresses a wistful romanticism. Unlike Phyllis, Monique admits to a preference for endowment, and a desire for experimentation—as well as openly and unfashionably admitting that there are times when she doesn't really like sex.

I am usually uncomfortable around men—there have been very few men in my life who have made me feel comfortable. Those men made me feel comfortable because they didn't expect me to live up to my image of the totally glamorous woman who is always made-up and manicured—that image does not coincide with myself inside. Most men don't realize that. I don't think I like sex as much as I thought I did. Sex doesn't really matter to me very much. It never did. I have orgasms with sex—but not like I think I should have; other women telling they have eight, nine, twelve, fourteen orgasms—but I'm really happy if I have one—*that's* an achievement. Anyway, you can have a lot of orgasms masturbating.

Does fantasizing and masturbating give you better orgasms than having sex with someone?

Yes. It's mental masturbation—I can have an orgasm by just thinking. I fantasize about certain men—I fantasize about Nureyev, who is my closest friend and lives here. The fact that I fantasize so much about certain men makes them very exciting.

Describe your fantasy man to me.

He is a mixture of Nureyev, Maximilian Schell, and Yul Brynner.

Do those men have any particular qualities in common that turn you on?

None of them are American. There is not one American man who turns me on. I do like the power of American men when they are in a high position—but I am not attracted to American men per se.

I think American men are very sexually experimental. But I have a passion for Slavic men.

So do I. Slavs know how to create romance—they have something wild about them. The best lover I've ever had was a Russian—very dark and handsome. I had the same excitement out of going to bed with him as a white woman must have when she goes to bed with a black man.

Would you like to go to bed with a black man?

No—not at all. I don't like black men—I am racist. In order for me to be excited by a man I've got to feel that he is superior to me, whether he is or not. Somehow I can't get turned on if I feel the man is inferior to me. I think that black people should be with black people. But I like Arab men. I think of the desert, a camel, being carried away to a tent. I always think that Arabs have oil wells, jewels—that they have a harem where I will be head girl. I've never been with a Jewish man; they say Jewish men are fantastic to their wives, but awful to their girlfriends.

What other qualities do Maximilian Schell, Nureyev, and Yul Brynner have in common?

They are masculine, intriguing. They are attracted to women without flopping all over them. They have a mystery about them—they seem remote, not available to the first woman who wants them. Yul was available to me—but he is not available to everyone. Yul has a great face, a great body, and a super mind. I love the way he is built—his immense shoulders and slender waist. He has great sexual appeal, but he is not a predator—he is not there to just conquer another woman. I like the combination of masculine and feminine in a man. I find David Bowie quite fascinating. Is he feminine? Is he masculine? I find something quite ambiguous about him which turns me on very much. I find the masculine man is not necessarily represented by all those muscles. I find David Bowie extremely masculine with his slim look. I can imagine going to bed with him.

Are there any men you would like to go to bed with but haven't?

Maximilian Schell—but I will. Fidel Castro. Kissinger was also quite appealing to me. I would have liked to with Brando. I like Engelbert Humperdinck—but not Tom Jones; he's too obvious.

My fantasy men are Gregory Peck, Zubin Mehta, General Dayan, Sinatra, Pierre Trudeau, and Richard Burton—I interviewed him yesterday and I think he's very sexy.

Not at all—I made a film with Elizabeth Taylor called *Ash Wednesday* in Venice. Richard Burton was very much after me—he was bold and said things like "Come upstairs and see the new Venetian glass I've bought," describing to me in detail how big he was. He didn't turn me on at all—I don't like unsubtlety.

What about Warren?

I like him.

You paused for a long time. What about Redford?

God no. He's not my type sexually—but I love him as an actor. Male stars don't turn me on. I went to bed with some men truly because their image was so super-sexy and I wanted to see what the sensation was all about—out of curiosity. Years ago I was friends with Elvis Presley—maybe he learned later, but to me the sex was a disaster. Just missionary-style—not interesting. I visited his mother in Memphis—I remember she gave me sausages and I pretended that I loved them, but I really didn't like them at all. Elvis used to send me them and thought he was doing me a great favor. I was very depressed when he died, especially when I heard about all the gifts he used to give those other girls, and all *I* ever got from Elvis was sausages from Memphis.

Was he very much a mother's boy?

Yes.

Did that make Elvis passive in bed?

No. He was very romantic, sent flowers, left me little notes, he was charming.

Do you think he was sexually very experienced?

No. He was just starting out. I don't think he had time to experiment. And when someone has such a reputation he can never live up to the expectation. I expected an earthquake—but it didn't happen. Famous women are under the same pressure—expected to be very sexual. So you wonder if you are living up to what they expect.

Do you ever worry whether a man wants you for yourself or for your image?

I never know—and I frankly don't care. I have to be truthful; how does one know if one is not attracted to a man because of his good looks, his reputation, his position in life? I suppose I feel that men with money and power can really have whatever they want. So if they choose you, it is truly because of their total interest in you as a person. Power in a man is terribly attractive.

How does power translate sexually? They say that men who have great power are submissive in bed. Have you found that?

Yes, absolutely—I am sure of it, from my experience.

Talking about experience, do you think experience makes a man better in bed?

I've always liked men in their forties—even when I was sixteen. I am not a pioneer, and I would rather someone else trained the boys. Men in their forties have already been through all the models and hat-check girls, so they want *you* because they want a woman. Every man I've ever really cared for was older than I. I've only cared for two men in my life that were younger. One of them died tragically in a car accident eighteen years ago—I was five years older than he—he was one of the great loves of my life. I find it more and more difficult to find men who appeal to me. I don't like men whom I know for a fact have had lots of women—who just go with a woman to put another number in their books. I don't want to be another number. But I do like strong men.

Give me your definition of a strong man.

A man who you know will look good in black leather—will know where to take you at night without asking, will know what wine to order without asking, will have tickets for a play instead of wondering where to go that night, will have air tickets to take you to a divine place for the weekend. In bed he is dominant—but I think that a man who is very dominant is much more of a slave in a sexual relationship than the one who carries the whip. Because the man who is subservient in bed is clearly the stronger of the two. Subservience lasts only as long as the one who is subservient wants it and not longer. You are not really the master of someone subservient—he is. But it doesn't necessarily have to be kinky.

What do you define as kinky?

Everybody is trying to get into S&M. I fantasize about it, but I've never experimented. I had a very Catholic upbringing which has always put barriers in my head. When I truly am in love with someone I can't do things with him that I've fantasized. My fantasies could only be had with people I'll never see again—but at the same time I am unable to have relationships with people I don't believe in. I wish I could be freer.

What else would you like to do?

Everything. I've never been to an orgy—I've only ever had very straight, normal relationships with men, without accouterments. But women fascinate me—especially the kind you see in porno magazines. But I don't like nude men in porno magazines.

Does a man have to be well endowed to be good in bed?

I like it. Women who say that size doesn't matter are bullshitting. To me it does. Some men like flat-chested women—other men like large breasts. I am the same about men.

How important is stamina—the length of time a man can have sex?

It's not important to me—because if sex goes on too long I get terribly bored and tired. At the beginning of a relationship I do want the sex to last forever, but after a while you know what to expect. Then I don't want the sex to go on for long—it bores me and I want something else.

What makes a man special for you?

A man is memorable if he woos me. If he makes me do things for him in a sexual sense and in my way of life that I wouldn't do for anyone else. A man should make a woman believe what she doesn't believe. He should build her up—so that if she is beautiful he should tell her; nothing works better than flowers and compliments. He should also be very generous. If he has money, he should spend it on a woman; if he is poor he can be generous with his time.

What advice would you give to men who want to be good in bed?

Don't go with little girls—you'll learn nothing from them, because they themselves are learning. But I've made mistakes in my life—I've always chosen the wrong man. I've always had the most complicated situations—either the man is married, or poor, or gay, and sometimes I hit the jackpot and they are all three. They say a man goes to bed with a woman for sex, hoping to find love, but a woman goes to bed with a man for love, hoping to find sex. I don't really feel that love is necessarily related to sex. But I always enter a new relationship with the feeling that "this is love."

Do you need the man to feel the same?

I always hope he will—and I always believe he does. But still, with the person you love you can't have the same wildness as you do when you know you may never see the man again. I am much shyer with someone I love. And when I am with a man I like, I always try to find a nightgown in my closet that has no story, no past, because at least the nightgown should be virginal—even if I'm not.

Sylvia Miles

Middle-aged actress Sylvia Miles is also an ex-Warhol star and social butterfly. In fact, I first met Sylvia at an Andy Warhol party, dressed in a long peasant dress, with silk flowers stuck in her long streaked hair. A few months later, I interviewed her at the Savoy in London before Sylvia was due to open in Tennessee Williams's *Vieux Carré*. Sylvia was nervous, so we set up another interview for after the opening. We met again in Sylvia's dressing room at the Piccadilly Theatre. There, surrounded by congratulation telegrams and cards from well-wishers, Sylvia was patently proud of her newly won stage success, dazzled that her name was up in lights in Piccadilly Circus.

A native New Yorker, Sylvia Miles nevertheless reminded me of Californians—with flowers permanently in her hair, Indian dresses, and frequent reference to "vibes." The keynote of Sylvia's interview is, "You can't separate sex from the rest of a relationship." She also comments on the differences between European and American men, from the viewpoint of a temporary European resident.

At the moment I am so involved with my life and my work that probably I don't have the same preoccupation with social or personal relationships as I had at one time. The press always teases me about being so social, such a party girl, always visible, but I've always been alone doing all those things and working. I've never had an entourage on location or anywhere, and the only time I've ever been part of a group was when I made *Heat* with Andy Warhol. Now I have totally and completely accepted the reality of what it means to be alone, and that I will perhaps be alone forever—for the rest of my life. But at the same time I feel more able to be with another human being because my relationships are no longer based on an inability to be alone.

What kind of a man do you think is able to cope with a career woman like yourself?

It seems to me that there is no one way in which a relationship works—and I haven't seen that relationships work better when one partner is not committed to a career. That has nothing to do with it all. I think respect makes relationships work. When two people respect each other and are aware of each other's uniqueness and individuality, there is no need to diminish or change one another. You can learn to appreciate and understand and live with someone who is different from you—and as long as you respect that difference the relationship will work. But relationships fall apart when one person expects the other to behave in a certain way.

How does that apply to sex?

You can't separate sex from the rest of a relationship. If there is too much expectation in sex, then one partner may feel cheated or violated or taken advantage of—which destroys respect.

How do you think each partner should communicate what they want?

Ideally you shouldn't have to communicate that at all. If you have to sit down and figure it out at any length, then obviously the person you are with is not that much in tune with you. Two people ought to want to do things for each other of their own volition. It rarely works if partners try to please the other and not themselves. Two people who try totally to please themselves will end up really pleasing each other.

What kind of an approach do you prefer from men?

I certainly don't find anything wrong with flattery. If I find a man attractive and I like him and he is flattering as well, that might win me. Men are different in England than in America. In England men are a bit more reserved—they like to think of it as being civilized, but to an American it's being less direct. Latin men tend to be more open and overt about wanting you and letting you know that they do. But that doesn't necessarily mean that the relationship will work out much better, or that the man won't react the same way to the next woman he meets ten minutes later.

What turns you off in a man?

Being ungraceful. But anything that is in good taste is okay. Good taste means right for that situation— within that relationship. If people are really in tune with each other they will know what is in bad taste— what is jarring or upsetting. It's like a play—you shouldn't be jarred out of the reality of that play; you have to believe in the other actor's moves. Nothing will really be jarring if it is heartfelt. You have to believe in the play and in the other actor—otherwise you shouldn't be appearing in that play with him. And the same applies to sex.

What advice would you give to a man who wants to be good in bed?

Use your brain. The more you use your brain, the better sex will be. Apply your intelligence to the sexual situation. And be like a good actor—believe in the play and give the characterization your whole heart and soul, and of course include the body as well!

Carroll Baker

Like Sylvia Miles, Carroll Baker is currently living in London, and talked to me about American men. When I interviewed Carroll in her Hampstead house she was on the verge of filming *The World Is Full of Married Men*. Her hair is white-blond, her skin is like porcelain, her eyes are china-blue, and her figure slim, so I was surprised to find the Carroll Baker of *Harlow*, *Baby Doll*, and *The Carpetbaggers* virtually unchanged. There is, however, one slight alteration: in blue jeans, white sneakers, and pink sweater, Carroll Baker was closer to cheerleader and outdoor girl than pin-up and sultry sex symbol.

Carroll Baker was crisp, efficient, formal, self-contained, but displayed sudden sparkles of irony as she parodied the American way of romance. She stabbed accurately at pretentious American men who instantly wanted "meaningful relationships." Her description of Italian men echoed Rossano Brazzi and Giancarlo Gianinni. But unlike Phyllis Diller, Regine, and Barbara Cartland, Carroll Baker doesn't expect to always have sex with love, and doesn't deride women's liberation, instead observing that "it is going to take ten to fifteen years before we really see the effects of women's liberation on men, as well as women."

I think there should be a lot of mystery about sex, and I don't like it to be too clinical because that spoils the mystery for me. And in a relationship I don't believe in overfamiliarity; I think—especially if you are living together—that each person should have his or her own privacy. When I go into the bathroom I don't want to leave the door open or anyone to come in—I just don't want that kind of familiarity.

You've lived in Europe for many years—do you find European sexual attitudes different from American ones?

Yes. I think there is an unrealistic romanticism that exists in America and is rarely present in Europe. Some English female friends of mine told me the other day that they had just met some American men and they asked me what I thought of American men. I told them that I get put off by all these American men who say, "Let's have a meaningful relationship." Everything immediately has to be so meaningful that you are instantly put off. Well, two days later I met my English friends again—they roared with laughter and one said, "Carroll, you'll never believe this, but I was arranging a date with an American man and the first thing he said to me was, 'I think we are going to have a meaningful relationship.' I laughed so much that I broke the date." I particularly like the Italian attitude. Italian men feel that a romance is a romance and that you are together because romance is wonderful—not because you expect something to be meaningful or to last a lifetime.

Erika Padan Freeman says that seasoned seducers always seduce women by promising them a lifelong relationship.

I think that is being very dishonest—and I think any woman with the slightest bit of experience will recognize the dishonesty. When you reach a certain age, and are both worldly, why not be honest if you are attracted to each other?

Do you think attraction is enough or do you need to love someone before you have sex with him?

Absolutely not. Sex is a physical need. But of course there is nothing greater than the combination of love and sex.

How has your attitude toward sex changed since you were a teenager?

As a young girl I was very influenced by that unrealistic American romanticism, mentioned before. So when I got married I believed my marriage would last forever. Then when we broke up, after twelve years, I had a nervous breakdown, through feeling guilty and that the divorce was my fault. When I was single again I wanted to have a good time—and I really stayed as far as possible away from any relationship that might have become remotely serious, because I felt that as my marriage failed so would my relationships. And if you are thirty-five and don't have a man of your own you don't wait till you find the big romance of your life, but look for small relationships here and there. So I merely had fun. But now I have a stable relationship.

Do you think women's liberation has changed relationships between men and women?

I think it is going to take ten to fifteen years before we really see the effects of women's liberation on men, as well as women. As far as sexual relationships are concerned, I don't think feminism has really settled. But Madison Avenue is certainly pushing it. So many TV ads are horrifying; they present the man as being weak, stupid, and very concerned about the brand of floor polish he uses. Inevitably he goes out and buys the wrong sort—then when he comes home his wife says, "This is the one you should *really* have." Whereupon he looks at her in amazement because she is so bright. I think that is terrible. I wouldn't give a second thought to a man who would even go and *buy* floor polish. And if he cared which brand *I* bought, I wouldn't talk to him again.

How do you feel about macho men?

To me "macho" means "muscle man." I'm into health and exercise myself, so I enjoy macho men who jog and do pushups. I made a film in Mexico and the Mexican actors were very macho, and I quite like that.

Is there any age group of man that you think is sexiest?

When I was about thirty-five I went through a stage when I dated younger men—but I've passed through that stage now. Most of my life I've preferred men who were my age—my husband was, and so is the man I am now with.

Do you have a type of man you prefer?

No—but I've never really been attracted to very, very handsome men. I think men who are very handsome are too involved with themselves and are always looking for their own reflection. Anyway, I've never wanted to go out with anyone prettier than me. But I did have a crush on Clark Gable. I was totally in love with him as a kid—then I got to make *But Not for Me,* and when Gable put his arms around me on the set I thought I'd faint. The film was late in his career and he had palsy, but Gable was still not a disappointment to me because he was such a wonderful human being.

You started your career with a very sexy image, because of Baby Doll. *Did your sex symbol image frighten men?*

I don't think it frightened them, but I did have one or two strange reactions. I've had a couple of men with problems who thought that maybe because I was a sex symbol I could solve their problems with some special formula I had. I was horrified. I said to this one man: "I don't mind at all being friends if you want to remain friends—but sex is out, because we are just incompatible." And he said, "Won't you have patience with me? You know I have problems." So I said, "Your problems are not my problems—why should I have patience?" Then he said, "But you are one of the great sex symbols—if you can't solve my problems, who can?" And I said, "A psychiatrist, my dear, a psychiatrist. I am just an ordinary woman."

What for you makes good sex?

I think it is very individual and very personal. The chemistry between two people is a mystery, like so much of nature, and can never be defined. We all grow up with fantasies about sex, and I believe that a good relationship fulfills those fantasies. So if you are fortunate enough to find someone who fulfills your fantasies, and if you fulfill his, then the sex will be good for both of you.

Diane Von Furstenberg

Elegant Belgian-born Diane Von Furstenberg talked to me in her Fifth Avenue office—newly decorated in feminine shell-pink and violet. I was intrigued to meet Diane, after having interviewed her estranged husband, Egon, and having read about her phenomenal success as a fashion designer. Diane wore a black dress and black boots with a white leather motif; her hair was long in loose curls and she had little makeup and no nail varnish—a departure, she later told me, from the original glossy Diane Von Furstenberg image.

Before the interview began, Diane asked whether I minded if she worked on her correspondence while we talked. I said no, so throughout the interview Diane sifted through letters, invitations, and press releases in a businesslike crisp way. I sat on the other side of the desk, feeling formal, as Diane answered my questions unfalteringly, promptly, and self-confidently in her throaty Belgian accent. Intelligent, feminine, and professional, Diane Von Furstenberg combines European mystique and femininity with American drive, freedom, and progressiveness.

A woman makes a man a good lover. The chemistry that turns a man into a good lover is being with a woman who is right for him. I think a woman should emphasize different things about herself with each man—which doesn't mean hiding other things. It is very exciting to be a woman. Part of the fun that I have is that I can always say, "Well, I am a woman," and be flirtatious and fun in situations where otherwise I should have to be extremely serious. I am very warm, I am extremely kind to men. I totally believe in giving men tenderness. I make men feel very good.

I believe a woman should flatter a man—I believe in making a man feel great, it doesn't cost anything. I strongly believe a woman should compliment a man, as long as the flattery isn't obnoxious or stereotyped. The worst thing one can do is to make someone feel he is being told the same thing as you have told someone else.

I also don't believe a man should necessarily make all the moves. It is a question of chemistry—and I don't see any reason why the woman shouldn't make the moves. There is no rule. Men are shyer than women, American men are even shyer than European men. American men are also more romantic—I don't think European men are as romantic. They are more outgoing, though; they will pick a woman up in the street very quickly and easily. They are also more possessive than American men.

I think American men are much nicer than European men. American men are much more cozy and less threatened by a woman than European men are. Women have always been much stronger in America—there is a pioneer inside every American woman. So American men are much more used to fighting alongside their women. I think all men are wonderful—I like men—but American men are men *par excellence*. They may have weaknesses, but they also have wonderful kindness, warmth, and generosity. They are very generous in giving of themselves. Sometimes, I think, American men are too nice and then women walk all over them.

I don't feel that men are threatened by a woman being intelligent. If a woman is intelligent she doesn't have to show off or prove to a man she is intelligent— she plays things very differently with each man. I know that from experience. When I started in fashion I was much more insecure, so I would put on a little bit of an air. I looked a lot harder than I really was—than I am now. I would wear bright lipsticks and bright nail varnish, and lots of mascara. But the wonderful thing that happens with success is that you can be yourself. It is easier to accept yourself when you have been accepted publicly by other people. Success means that you can be who you are. Sometimes people are slightly intimidated. The other day I met someone, and later he told me, "If I had known who you were . . ." You have a wonderful conversation with someone, when they find out who you are and they freak.

The most important thing is to be comfortable with yourself, to be in control of your life. But not too much in control. You should always leave room for the unexpected, which is always the most exciting. It's nice sometimes not to decide, especially if you are a woman—you want sometimes not to decide. There is the thought of something that is a little dangerous, or unexpected. The unexpected is the most beautiful. I think one of the most exciting things is meeting people you are not supposed to meet—people who are out of your context. Because then you can move away from yourself, so probably live out your fantasies. But I think that one's fantasies are very much one's own. You want to live them out, but your fantasies are very personal, and I don't think a man should try to find them out; they will either develop instinctively or they won't.

But you probably can't have everything from one man—each person will give you something else. Sometimes I've had wonderful close relationships, but you are still two different people. I think the success of a relationship is two people remaining individuals. I don't think anyone changes another person, though, but people should try to influence one another.

I have discovered that I am terribly maternal—I always look at men in a very understanding way. I never discard anyone once a sexual relationship is over. I understand and respect people—therefore if a man ceases to love me, I guess I can understand that too. It's never really happened—not with someone who really cared for me—with little quick affairs, yes, but otherwise not. And once someone has been in my life, they will always be in my life. My family is getting bigger and bigger as the years go by, because I will always love someone I love, although the love may change. When the chemistry is there, it is wonderful—and when it is no longer there, I think that all you can say is that it was wonderful, and it evolved into something that is different but equally wonderful. I have never stopped being good friends with someone once I have stopped having sex with them. I am capable of having sex with someone, then no longer having sex, but still loving him all the same.

I will tell my children that giving love is never wrong, but that respecting yourself is more important—the most important thing is to be responsible for yourself, and to make right judgments. I love relationships, I love meeting people, I love talking to them and finding out about their craziness. I am very free and independent, and being free is not being limited, not having rules or preconceived ideas. I am very honest and open, there are no rules, and whatever happens in a relationship, in love and sex, just happens.

Debbie Harry

Debbie Harry has been labeled the Marilyn Monroe of rock. "Blondie" lead singer and '70s sex symbol Debbie was mobbed by press and fans at the London reception where I first met her. We talked again a few days later, in the garden of the Gloucester Hotel, where Debbie had just finished interviews with a stream of journalists. Dressed in a black silk see-through shirt, jeans, and sneakers, she answered my questions uninhibitedly. Perhaps a rarity among female rock singers, Debbie Harry was polite and professional.

I asked Debbie Harry about the supposedly wild world of rock, and her attitude to men is predictably basic. She says an orgasm is very important to her and that "more than likely I wouldn't bother with a man again if he didn't make me come." When I showed Debbie's interview to another female star she said, "Now *that* is *macho*." Debbie Harry is far too glamorous for such a masculine label—shouldn't someone invent a feminine equivalent?

In my teens all I wanted was a cute boyfriend who turned me on and took me out. I never really thought about who or what I wanted in bed. My mother was very liberal and educated me about sex, but she didn't encourage me to have any before marriage—because it just wasn't done. So I followed the rules of the dating game—you had a boyfriend, or lots, and you went out on dates. You ran the gamut, then after a while you either got bored with dating, but still went on doing it, or you settled down with one person. But I think that attitudes to sex in America have changed since I grew up because of the Pill. Women find it easier to have sex now.

Do you think men care if women want them just for sex?

No. When you are out meeting guys, sex is usually the mutual object. If I am going to have a one-night stand just for sex and someone comes on to me, I say, "Let's go make out, get laid, fuck, or whatever." If I want to—or I tell him to piss off if I don't. It depends on me—it has nothing to do with the man, it depends on what I feel like. But the man might still be upset if I, after a successful evening, am no longer attracted to him and he wants a repeat performance.

Do you ever feel you have to live up to a sexy image in bed—to actually "perform"?

Occasionally you do feel you have to put on a show in bed—but that really depends on the man you are with. Sometimes I just go along with it whatever it is.

Do you get male groupies?

I have been involved with Chris for two years—but I do get a lot of male groupies. Lots of them are fabulous—I've got one in California who sends me bouquets of flowers every night, which is really flattering. And I've had the chance to go out with some stars.

How do you like a man to approch you before bed?

Nowadays I think that sexual compatibility is easier to find than friendship. So the most successful approach to a woman, which most men ignore, is a disarming one; a way of approaching her out of simple friendship and acquaintanceship, as if they are trying to be your friend. Some men are direct—but I don't like the macho approach. I am not attracted to macho men, and I don't have much experience of them, but I think that their attitude—that men are always superior—is unnatural.

People may imagine that rock stars are very wild. What shocks you sexually?

Bestiality would shock me—but luckily no one has ever suggested it to me.

Do you think drugs make good sex?

I think drugs do sometimes make sex easier because they free your inhibitions.

Do you think a man should ask a woman what she wants sexually?

Yes—definitely. Or if he doesn't, the woman should still try to say something like "Look—this isn't happening—do you want to try this? It really turns me on." But if you are too shy to say that and the man doesn't ask you what you want, you just have to forget and try and enjoy what he *is* giving you—what is actually happening.

Does it matter to you if a man brings you to orgasm?

I think that is really important. More than likely I wouldn't bother with a man again if he didn't make me come. Even though I do think there is too much emphasis on the orgasm in American men's magazines, I am glad that it is fashionable now for men to be aware of the woman's orgasm. So that they remember that women have a clitoris and it's more than just a fuck. I think in four or five years' time every man will remember that automatically and really concentrate on the women he goes to bed with. Lack of concentration makes a man awful in bed.

What makes a man good in bed?

It's not any one thing, or a set of things—it's the total. Personality is important, and I also think men should let themselves be feminine, more sensual, and show their emotions. I like a man who is eager to laugh in bed—either at himself or at me, or at an ironic situation like the phone ringing or the bed falling down. Sometimes you can have a terrible time with a guy, then the next time it can be great—go on and on—so you don't think of anything else the next day. You can make out with somebody all the way through, but it still doesn't happen, you aren't satisfied, and you think, "Well—is it happening or not?" Then afterward you suddenly get a great feeling like you do when you drink a wine with a terrific, unforgettable aftertaste.

Cheryl Tiegs

I interviewed Californian Cheryl Tiegs, the world's number-one model, at the Sherry-Netherland Hotel in New York. That week *Time* magazine was following her everywhere for a cover story, and Cheryl was in New York for a series of interviews, of which mine was one. She was courteous and cautious, and I could tell that whenever Cheryl answered a question she was also judging how it would be received. Shrewd, pretty even without makeup, Cheryl Tiegs obviously carefully weighs the consequences of her words—so that when I submitted the interview for her approval she cut some of her more controversial comments. Even though she was circumspect, Cheryl was still honest enough to discuss having sex for attraction and not love.

Like Monique Van Vooren and Phyllis Diller, Cheryl doesn't value stamina in a man, and like Monique Van Vooren, Cheryl Tiegs allows that there are times when she doesn't really feel like sex.

I was glad to get a female view of sex in America in the '50s, and I also like Cheryl's comments on men in Hollywood. She was friendly, giggled a lot, gossiped about men we knew in Hollywood, and sometimes was unwittingly earthy.

I'm glad that I grew up in the '50s and '60s because sex was a bit slower in those days—you didn't just jump into bed at fourteen or fifteen. It was a big deal to kiss or touch somebody; we'd go to parties, play Spin the Bottle, give someone a big kiss, and that was it. When I was in high school there was a lot of dating and necking in cars, and at sixteen or seventeen we would kiss for hours, just lying with each other and not really having sex. Then the revolution of the '60s brought about a freedom of thinking; whatever you wanted to do was all right, as long as it made you happy and didn't hurt anyone else.

I've always been attracted to my opposite; my husband is very dark and tall and handsome and mysterious. He was at the top of his profession when I met him—but he never said anything about it, there was a quietness about him. I would never have gone out with a man who had a very loud boisterous voice, because that would be part of his personality.

I can't answer your question about the five men I would most like to go to bed with. I know most of the men in your book. Some of the men who are sexy on screen are just as sexy off—but others aren't. The film business is very sophisticated—and actors have girls knocking on their doors constantly. I suppose famous actors must feel that they have a reputation to live up to every time they go to bed. But they create that reputation; they don't have to go to bed with all those girls.

I don't remember ever going to bed with somebody I wasn't really attracted to and didn't want to see a lot. I have to be attracted to a man both mentally and physically. But sometimes you can be very attracted to a man but still say no. There could be many reasons why you refused, and the man shouldn't take it personally. Even within a relationship there are periods when I feel very sexy and periods when I don't. There are periods I go through when I am working too hard— I'm too busy, too preoccupied, and just don't feel like sex. I'm sure it's the same for the man—and neither of you should take it as a rejection.

Men will come on to you if you let them. I put on a cold exterior sometimes when I am working—if you are too open the man assumes things. So I walk into the studio, go about my business, or read a book—then nobody approaches me. It is up to the woman. I don't like it when men look you up and down—they are just trying too hard. And I think the worst approach is cliché'd lines like "Oh, you are the most beautiful, fascinating girl I've ever seen—I'd give up anything for you." I'm sure they say that to every girl—an attitude. A look is always better than a verbal approach.

I like a man who is a little soft in his approach—not really coming on to me, just being with me, having a nice time, so things happen naturally. The thing that turns me on most is kindness. I absolutely melt if a man is kind to me. Sincerity is also one of the most important things, and I can tell in a second if it is genuine. I can recognize the men who are putting on an act—I think men should just be themselves.

Even though a man might be lovely and sexy and attractive, he may not be good in bed. And the first time you have sex is not necessarily the best. You are both discovering each other. You are both trying to figure out what the other person likes, and that takes several times. When you have learned about the other person, I think the sex becomes better. I don't like men who try to find out what you like verbally. It just happens by not saying anything, by not talking about it—just by being very sensitive. I don't think a woman has to tell a man what she likes—if he does something she likes he will know it by the way she reacts. I think you have to verbalize fantasies; otherwise you will never discover your partner's—whether you like fantasies, whether you have ever had them. But I think fantasies are fantasies and should not be realities. I think fantasies and dreams are what they are and shouldn't be carried out.

I don't think a man is automatically great in bed if he goes on and on for ages. In fact, some of the most exciting times are when you just do it in five minutes. That can be just as sexy as going on for three hours. If I had to advise a man on how to be good in bed, I would tell him to be gentle. I like a man who is very sensitive to what I would like, just as I would try to be

with him. To spend an evening, get to know a man. I
love to touch and feel and kiss. The most important
thing is when the man totally concentrates on me, and
makes me feel that he has forgotten everything else in
the world except me.

Geraldine Chaplin

CHARLIE CHAPLIN: What do you want to be when you
grow up?

WENDY: I want to be an actress.

CHARLIE CHAPLIN: Be an actress, my dear, but never,
never marry an actor.

I was six years old, sitting on Charlie Chaplin's
knee in the Elizabethan dining room at Great
Fosters Hotel, England, when Chaplin gave me
that advice. And I took some of it; although I
never did become an actress, I also never married
an actor. The closest I came was that same afternoon when I played bride and Charlie's son
Michael, later an actor, played groom. I still have
the photograph of us all, standing in the porch of
Great Fosters. I wore a veil, Michael held my
arm, and Geraldine, Josie, and Vicki were our
bridesmaids, and underneath twelve-year-old
Michael Chaplin wrote, "To my bride Wendy."
I first met the Chaplin children when my
parents took me to a tea at Great Fosters. I
played with some children in a sandpit, and one
of them, Vicki Chaplin, gave me a little doll, and
took me to meet her father, Charlie. I had never
heard of him, but became friends with Vicki, who
was my age. A few months later I was invited to
stay with the Chaplins at their lakeside home in

Vevey, Switzerland. After dressing me primly and properly in frills and lace, my parents deposited me at the door of the Chaplins' gracious mansion. Vicki and I then spent the entire day sitting on the wall surrounding the estate, throwing mud and stones at all the tourists who came to gape at Charlie Chaplin's home. Until Kay-Kay and Pinney, the Chaplin nannies, discovered us covered in mud and grass, and sent us straight to bath and bed. As a result, fifteen-year-old Geraldine was charged with chaperoning us, whereupon she protected us from being "caught" during midnight feasts and more mud-throwing. I discovered that although life with the Chaplins seemed outwardly opulent, especially to outsiders, it was in reality simple, average, and fun.

Somehow I lost touch with the Chaplins—so when I phoned Geraldine nearly twenty years later, after hearing she was in Beverly Hills, she was understandably flabbergasted to find that the "little Wendy" she remembered had become a "sex-book" authoress. We met for tea, laughed about the past, and promised to keep in touch. A year later, again in Beverly Hills, Geraldine aptly became my first female interviewee for *What Makes a Man G.I.B.*

Geraldine was very articulate, and although she said, "I should have thought about this before," she obviously has strong beliefs about relationships. Her life-style is progressive; unmarried, she has a son, Shane, by Spanish director Carlos Sauras, and says categorically that she doesn't believe in monogamy. While Shane, a lovely little boy with huge brown eyes, played in the background, Geraldine, very slim in a navy boiler suit, sat on the floor as we talked. Despite her belief in polygamy, Geraldine said she wouldn't go to bed with a man she didn't love, for that moment—then proceeded to give her definition of love. She talked at length about men who turn sex into a stage production, and the ways in which her attitudes to relationships have changed since she was a teenager. And although time and friendship may perhaps prejudice me, I think that Geraldine Chaplin, intelligent, free, and feminine, is the consummate "new woman" the experts talk about.

I hate men who are very conscious of their sexual performance—who want to create an impression in bed—who think, "I am good—I am going to create a memory in this lady—boy, is she going to remember me." I hate that. I feel instinctively when men are like that—it's almost like a live sex show; you feel as if you are watching it and you know that the man is thinking, "This is what I should do, and this and this and that."

American men have a fixation about being good in bed—about being a good lay. Experience makes me say that; I had an affair with a man that went on for a long time, but we couldn't go to bed because he was married. When we finally got to bed, he was terrified that his performance wouldn't be good. I think that is typical of American men—perhaps because American women are demanding and create a complex in men about being good in bed. None of that is important to me—it didn't matter to me at all—but it did to that man.

Every man I've been to bed with has been the right man at that moment—and the best. I've had men who were physical disasters—but that didn't matter, because they were the right man for that moment. If I had to tell a man how to be good in bed I would tell him to be good out of bed too. Erotic atmosphere is the clue to it all. I've had affairs with men who took me out to dinner and did a whole stage production of "I picked this caviar especially for you," told me things like "I am very sexual *and* very romantic," then as the grand finale, got me into bed, and tried to live up to all those things they told me at dinnner. Always I, I, I—

never giving. I think sex should be the prolongation of a nice conversation at dinner and eating well.

I don't believe in monogamy—in one man. I think sex has been made into more than it is by literature and magazines. It's antique to think that sex is something forbidden, or something sinful, or something wonderful. It's not—it's part of life, and going to bed with someone isn't really that important at all.

I don't see bed as the ultimate goal. I did have a phase in my life when I would go to bed with a man—then that would be the end of the relationship. It was like the Cinderella story—"They got married and lived happily ever after"—but now I no longer feel that bed is the first or last step in a relationship.

Sometimes you can look at a man, hug him, know you like him, and then, as far as I am concerned, you've already been to bed with him—the moment that you know you will, it's an unspoken agreement, chemistry. You like each other, so you know you are going to bed—because you fancy each other. But there are other times you may go to bed with someone and *not* go to bed with him—and there are other times you may go to bed with someone whom you don't fancy, just because the moment is right. Going to bed with an old friend can also be very nice—if a situation arises where you are alone together and go to bed—then it's nice and warm and affectionate. And sometimes having dinner with a man can be as sensual as going to bed with him.

I've never felt just physical lust for someone and just wanted him for that reason. I've always had a crush on someone—so going to bed was the natural consequence of that crush. I don't even notice a man's approach to me, I am so blinded by him. The thing that makes me want to go to bed with a man has to do with me. I don't care whether a man wants me for myself or for my image—the only thing I care about is if I want him and he wants me.

If I could create the ideal man in bed he would

probably be different every couple of months—a man
who changes. I would never demand anything in bed,
because I think if sex is going to go right, then it's going to go right. If the man acts out the role he wants to
act in bed—and that is the role I want him to act—
then everything will be fine. Things like sex don't really
mean a thing—to me sex is a question of giving.

I couldn't go to bed with a man I didn't love—for
that moment. To me love and sex must always be
related. I may love somebody for five minutes—but I
definitely love a man when I go to bed with him. And
the man who is good in bed loves me for that moment
and thinks that I am attractive and really likes me. I
don't think it matters whether all that is real or not—
just as long as I, for that moment, believe it. And I
think the worst thing a man can do in bed is to say
something about a woman's looks—that she's too fat
or too thin.

Men are always afraid to say, "I love you," but I say
"I love you" to anyone I love at that moment. All
those centuries of Christianity have deceived us into
thinking that love is permanent. But love isn't permanent. Love is never permanent—it goes through a
lot of changes. One day it's love in this way, then love
in that way, then love in this way, then sexual love,
then romantic love, then another kind of love. Love is
never the same for every moment, with every person,
never the same with the same person. You go through
a stage with someone when you are terribly horny for
them, then that may taper off, and happen again later,
or never happen again, but you may still love them or
you may not.

Making love can also be a matter of power. Usually
a relationship in bed establishes itself early on, with
one person having power over the other. And if you
are in bed with someone who is younger or less experienced than you are, you naturally adopt the power
role. But both a man and a woman should be able to
relinquish power in bed—to give up needing to have

someone under their spell. Because the greatest relationships happen when power no longer exists, when you are no longer trying to be the most attractive, the best in bed he has ever had, and he is not trying to be the most attractive and the best lover you've ever had.

Shelley Duvall

Shelley Duvall and Geraldine Chaplin are both well known for their appearances in Robert Altman's films. I interviewed Shelley in the Dorchester Hotel, London, where she was filming Stanley Kubrick's *The Shining* with Jack Nicholson. We talked for three hours in her suite, ate salmon sandwiches, and compared notes on Hollywood and men. A few months later I sent Shelley a copy of her interview, and she edited it and returned it to me, complete with additional frank remarks on love, sex, and relationships. In her late twenties, Shelly, bright and articulate, is the youngest female interviewee in the book.

Shelley Duvall discusses promiscuity, orgies, verbal approaches, age groups and types of men, and the female orgasm, and she may surprise some men by focusing on the challenge which some women feel when the man they are with cannot get an erection. Shelley Duvall ("I think sex is for pleasure and fun and release—as well as children") is far removed in attitude from Barbara Cartland, who began this section.

I was very naive about sex until the first time I made love. I was sixteen years old and had never seen a man nude, nor had any encounters with a penis. I was very much a childlike teenager and looked at sex as something adults did when they were in love or wanted a child. Romance, kissing, and petting were all I was concerned about that night. It was my birthday and he was my first boyfriend. We were very drunk on champagne in the back seat of a '57 Chevy parked on a dark street. It was his second time. I remember we laughed a lot and had a good time. I still enjoy sex best with someone I like a lot and am attracted to.

Did that first sexual experience live up to your expectations?

I really didn't have any expectations about the first time. I am not a worrier by nature, and the event just sort of sneaked up on me. I was very happy being kissed and cuddled. Sex was never really discussed around our household, and the girls at school who had "done it" kept their secret well. It was a nice surprise.

Do you believe that love and sex always need to be related?

It's wonderful when they are, but I definitely don't think they need to be to have good, uninhibited sex. Love is more difficult to find. Sex is always available; *good* sex requires you to be more selective. I consider myself the more selective type. Promiscuity brings too many disappointments, and occasionally VD and that doesn't interest me at all.

Does sex always have to develop out of a relationship for you?

No, I've had sex with a stranger before, and it was good. I never saw him again, and it's not important to me that I ever do. It was very exciting. I don't view sexual encounters as events. I just enjoy the variations that come my way.

What is your definition of "promiscuous"?

I've never been to an orgy, and if I did go to one, I would have to be attracted to everyone involved, because to me promiscuity is having sex with people to whom you are not attracted. I'll make love to someone if I'm attracted to him and like him well enough.

Are you ever disappointed by sex?

Yes, sometimes, usually when I'm preoccupied with something or someone else and shouldn't have had sex in the first place. If I'm not feeling well, I sometimes just prefer to be cuddled. It's also disappointing when the man doesn't "give" much and you are in the mood for receiving.

Do you like it if a man asks you to go to bed with him?

It depends on how the line is delivered. I don't like to be libidinized by a libertine. Usually, the less verbosity, the more amatory the approach. It depends on the person, too. If it's someone you enjoy talking to, I usually find a good conversation part of a good flirtation. Other times it's more erotic when less is said. But the right man can do or say anything. It's still a matter of chemistry. It's important to me to be comfortable with the man, in and out of bed.

You mean relaxed—but when you used the word "comfort" I suddenly pictured one of those playboy singles apartments in L.A.

I once rented a house like that. There were little nude dolls that resembled the owner, and red lights in the bedroom. If I were led into a room like that I would probably laugh. I'd try to conceal it, but I would laugh. A good imagination and some good fantasies are all you need.

Do you have a type of man that you find especially sexy?

No. It's on an individual basis. The last time I had a type was as a teenager when I liked beach-boy types with blue eyes, chiseled features, and skin and hair very different from mine.

Like Ken of Barbie and Ken?

No, Ken was tall and thin and didn't have a penis. It seems I have a particular liking for Jewish men. Three out of four relationships were Jewish. I remember my mother telling me, "Jewish men make loyal husbands." She had no idea I'd have a career of my own, that I'd be married, divorced, and happy having adventures. It takes an intelligent and interesting man to keep me interested for a length of time, and those men are usually older than I am by eight to twelve years.

I've always preferred men fifteen to twenty years older than I—so I find it strange that some men like Egon and Rossano were seduced when they were ten by women of our age group.

I've never really been attracted to younger men, maybe because I have three younger brothers. I like the man to be as smart as I am and more worldly. That is not to say that all older men meet those standards. But they have had more practice than younger men, and tend to have more finesse. Maybe that was what those boys liked about the older women.

Do you think experience makes a man better in bed?

It helps, but there are many other factors—sensitivity, imagination, desire, ethos, all the inherent qualities that cannot be learned from books. Although sharing ideas does increase curiosity.

How do you think a man should discover what you want in bed?

I would show him what I like best during intercourse, or ask him to do it. I do to him what I'd like done to me. He can do whatever he likes to me, as long as there's no real pain or danger or animals, and if he likes what I'm doing better then he'll switch to that, or vice-versa. Fantasies are an important part of sex for me. When a fantasy is mutual, I think the orgasm is better for both. Speaking during sex is nice, too.

Men are now very aware of the female orgasm—"Did you come?" An actress I once interviewed said she felt like one of Pavlov's dogs, having to salivate when the bell rings.

I don't like being asked if I came. Sometimes I do and sometimes I don't come, just like men. Sometimes I come many times. That's part of all the variations that make it interesting, surprising. I don't place so much importance on whether or not the man comes, and I don't like being asked if I came as if I wouldn't enjoy it if I didn't. But I think men ask for themselves, for reassurance. They care about you and don't want to let you down either. Some women have stressed the importance of their orgasm to the point of frightening men. I think sex is best when played by ear—when you are dealing with the present moment, and feel free of inhibitions.

Do you think a man can tell if you have come?

I think a lot of men can't tell unless you are very verbal about it, and I don't like to say the words "I'm coming" when I'm lost in feeling. I don't say anything I don't feel like saying. Most of the time I can't speak when I am coming.

Do you like macho men?

Macho men can be very sexy sometimes. They are really a fantasy I've lived out a couple of times. I'm slightly masochistic, and they are a wonderful fantasy. I wouldn't get involved with a macho man, though. I prefer not to be held in jealousy; not to be restrained. Although I do like a man to dominate me to a degree.

Has the women's liberation movement affected your relationship with men?

No, I always considered myself to be free and equal and was very lucky never to have a confrontation with a man who felt otherwise.

What would you say to a man who asked your advice on how to be good in bed?

I would say to follow your instincts, be selective about the persons you choose to go to bed with, use your imagination, work on your inhibitions, be more unrestrained with your fantasies, think about the woman's pleasure, touch, caress, and lose yourself in ecstasy. Don't think about being "better," because *there is no failure.* A man can even be unable to get an erection and still be great in bed, a satisfying lover.

Do you think lack of size makes a man terrible in bed?

Size really doesn't matter. It's talent and sensitivity that count. I've been to bed with men who've had large penises and didn't know how to use them well. Most men would be surprised to hear how important the caresses and foreplay are to women. I don't mind if a man can't get an erection—I enjoy the foreplay; it's a challenge; it makes me excited to try. And if the man still can't get a hard-on after I've tried, it just makes the prospects greater for the next day. Drugs, alcohol, cigarettes, lack of sleep, stress, any of these things could be the cause, and none of these have long-lasting effects. You can just lie there and play all night. It can be just as pleasant and satisfying. I think sex is for pleasure and fun and release—as well as children. It's magic—and it's the magic that keeps us all interested.

SUMMARY OF
WHAT MAKES A MAN GOOD IN BED

1. Being sensitive and caring.
2. Mutual telling.
3. Telling the woman he loves her when he orgasms.
4. Treating the woman like a lady.
5. Bringing the woman to orgasm.
6. Simultaneous orgasms.
7. Stamina is unimportant. ?
8. Exciting the woman.
9. Skin.
10. Being dominant.
11. Having power.
12. Being well endowed.
13. Wooing the woman.
14. Flattering the woman.
15. Being intelligent.
16. Fulfilling the woman's fantasies.
17. Taking his time.
18. Building up a romantic feeling.
19. Treating the woman like a friend.
20. Laughing in bed.
21. Creating an erotic atmosphere out of bed.
22. Being changeable.
23. Loving the woman.
24. Thinking the woman is attractive and really liking her.
25. Giving up power in bed.
26. Not trying to be the best lover the woman has ever had.
27. Being soft in his approach.
28. Being dominant, strong, and possessive.
29. Being kind.
30. Concentrating totally on the woman.
31. Being sincere.
32. Being attractive mentally and physically.
33. Making the woman feel comfortable.
34. Acting out fantasies.

36. Remembering that sex is for fun.
37. Being a man who relaxes the woman.

SUMMARY OF
WHAT MAKES A MAN BAD IN BED

1. Wham, bang, thank you ma'am.
2. Not taking sexual instruction from a woman.
3. Having a lot of women and just treating each one like another number.
4. Going on too long so the sex becomes boring and tiring.
5. Expecting too much.
6. Trying to please the woman and not himself.
7. Being ungraceful.
8. Thinking in terms of conquering.
9. Being rough, verbally or physically.
10. Being macho.
11. Not making the woman orgasm.
12. Not communicating.
13. Being very conscious of his own sexual performance.
14. Commenting adversely on the woman's looks.
15. Looking the woman up and down before bed and trying too hard.
16. Coming on with cliché'd lines.
17. Verbalizing too much.
18. Asking the woman what she would like him to do in bed.
19. Asking the woman if she has had an orgasm.
20. Asking how he can be good in bed.
21. Wanting to play the female role.
22. Thinking he doesn't have to do anything.
23. Continually trying to make the woman orgasm.

Some men may be disturbed by the criticisms women made in this section, so for men who want to learn more about male sexuality, the next section consists of interviews with male hookers and superstuds on their sexual tricks and techniques.

Part IV

Hookers and Superstuds

This section is not for everyone. The language is sometimes crude, and the techniques basic—but for the curious, the hookers and the superstuds provide unparalleled advice and titillation.

Interviewee Selection

Before interviewing male hookers and superstuds, I talked to four female hookers on what their unusually vast experience had taught them about men. Next I talked to Harry Reems and John Holmes—porno stars respectively renowned for *Deep Throat* and endowment. Then I interviewed three male prostitutes for women. I like the idea of male prostitution; I *want* to be able to send for "room service" and to occasionally have sex without complications. Some women already do; male prostitution is flourishing in Las Vegas. When I discussed this with women of my age, many of them agreed that male prostitution might be desirable, fantasizing about male hookers and the quality of sex money can buy for adventurous women. Some men I told were curious and insecure about male hookers, others were inflamed and excited by the idea, speculating whether or not they could make the grade. So, for women who fantasize about having, and for men who fantasize about being, I talked to male prostitutes about their tricks, their techniques, and their profession.

Topics Discussed

Apart from discussing specific sexual techniques and skills, both the hookers and the superstuds talked about how to recognize the female orgasm (a problem focused on by both experts and celebrities), how women have changed since the sexual revolution, and the mechanics of being a male sex object. Some of the interviewees express contempt for women, others seem to have studied them, and the only common denominator is that <u>all the interviewees in this section stress the</u> <u>importance of giving a woman oral sex.</u>

Questions to Interviewees

How old were you when you first had sex?
How did you feel about your first sexual experience?
Do you think you were born sexual?
What was your sex life during your teens?
How did you learn to have sex?
? How did you learn sexual rhythm?
Has experience made you better?
How did you learn to hold back from orgasm?
How can you recognize the female orgasm?
Is it important for you to make a woman orgasm?
Why is it important for you?
How do you judge the sexuality of a woman before bed?
How do you find out what turns a woman on?
How do you discover her fantasies?
How would you advise a man to ask a woman to go to bed in noncommercial sex?
How would you advise a man to find out what a woman wants?

How do you persuade a woman to do something she has never done before?

Do you find women are more aggressive sexually nowadays?

Do you ever feel pressure to perform sexually?

Are you always ready to have sex?

Do you always enjoy sex?

Have you ever felt sexually inadequate?

What shocks you sexually?

Have you ever made sexual mistakes?

What advice do you have for men who want to be good at oral sex?

What is your general advice on being a good lover?

How does being in love affect your sexual perform-ance?

Why did you become a hooker?

What age group of women do you see?

Is there a type of woman who pays for sex?

Why do you think women pay for sex?

What kind of fantasies do the women have?

✓How do you excite yourself so you can have sex with a woman whose appearance repels you?

✓ How do you fake orgasm?

✓ How many times a night can you make love?

How has being a male prostitute altered your non-commercial relationships with women?

A Hooker Symposium

This interview is an amalgamation of conversa-tions with four Las Vegas hookers—sort of a hookers symposium—with the answers stream-lined into one interview. All four women have been working for over six years and have had sex with thousands of men. I wasn't undertaking one of those pseudoscientific surveys, but just wanted to discover what the unusually extensive experiences of these women had taught them about men. Although the situations in which these experiences were gained were commercial, and outside the context of relationships, I felt that the number of their experiences still qualify the hookers to pronounce on male sexuality.

I started by broaching a subject men worry about and women whisper over: pre-bed clues to male sexuality. A delicate way of asking if there are any outward signs of endowment before a man undresses—and according to the hookers, there are. Relating to the "experts," I asked the "experienced" about male sexual problems they had encountered. Then we talked about the relationship between a man's age and his sexuality, his profession and his sexuality (leading to bad news for athletes, gamblers, and powerful men). Next I asked the hookers—time-honored takers of male virginity—how they teach a virgin to have sex. We also discussed problems men have in recognizing the female orgasm and how they can. I ended by asking the women what makes them orgasm, and what makes a man good in bed for a multi-experienced hooker. It could, of course, be argued that hookers have little experience of male sexual prowess, because the men who go to bed with hookers on a professional basis (like stars who go to bed with groupies) don't bother about the woman or their own "performance." However, my interviews indicate that this is not always so; hookers have told me that many of their clients concentrate obsessively on bringing them to orgasm, and I once interviewed a young, handsome, famous divorcé who told me that now he has sampled everyone and everything, his greatest thrill, the highest sexual accolade, is "making" a jaded hooker orgasm.

Do you ever get any clues about a man's sexuality before you go to bed with him?

I can tell how big a man's penis is before he undresses or has a hard-on. I look at his ears; if the ear lobe hangs free, is not pinned to the side of a man's head, then I know that his penis is long. And if the ridge on the edge of a man's ear is big, then his penis will be big in circumference. Looking at a man's ears is the only reliable way of telling beforehand what a man's penis will be like. Build and height are very deceptive; sometimes short men are built like Tarzan and tall, big men don't have anything at all. Usually, though, fat men are very small. When they were slimmer they may have been well built—but as soon as they became fatter their cock sank into the area around it so that it looked smaller. I can also tell a lot about a man beforehand by watching the way in which he approaches me. If his hands shake and tremble, I know I have got trouble, but if he is self-confident, knows what he wants, and acts as if he is in charge, then he will be all right. Often, though, a man has to get to know a woman before he feels at ease with her. I can usually tell the first few times whether or not a man is a good lover. Of course, a man can always learn to be better. I see men who are now good lovers but weren't before I taught them by saying things like "Don't do that," "That hurts," "It doesn't feel good when you do that."

Is there any relationship between a man's age and his sexuality?

Men of forty and over are best in bed. Eighteen may be a man's sexual peak in terms of the number of climaxes, the strength of his erection, and how often he can make love—but most guys of eighteen are in too much of a hurry, they are selfish and go to bed with a woman for themselves. But men of forty have learned about women, they are more mellow, more gentle, don't come too quickly, and take the time to really satisfy a woman.

Is there any relationship between a man's profession and his sexuality?

Yes. Athletes usually come as soon as they put it in. They are bad lovers because their entire body is tuned toward their muscles. Gamblers are also bad lovers because they are only interested in making money—and when they lose they are likely to become masochistic, wanting to be punished sexually for having lost. Doctors are usually good lovers because they understand anatomy and don't hold your legs over your head because they can understand why that hurts a woman. Divorce lawyers are also excellent because they've had a lot of experience through playing around with so many clients. Powerful, successful men are bad lovers because they only want to be pleased—all they care about is their own orgasm. They just jump on a woman, come, jump off—and then expect her to tell them how great they were. Powerful, successful men couldn't care less about the woman they are in bed with because they know there is another one waiting in line. Also men who have a lot of people working for them, under their control, want to repeat that relationship in bed and are sadistic to a woman. Italians are also lousy lovers, because they have a reputation of being such great lovers—so they have nothing else to prove.

What kind of things do the men you see worry about?

Every time I unzip a man's pants he says, "Is mine big or is it little? Is it average?" They ask me how I rate the size of their penis—small or large? If it is small I don't tell them—but if it's a fairly good size I do. Men always worry about size. I don't think that size makes much difference. Men with big cocks often just jump on me and play horse. Lots of men with big cocks think all they need to do is get it in—then a woman will go wild. If a man is too big he can jab at you too hard and you can develop kidney problems. And if a man is too wide he doesn't have too much mobility; you can't tense or tighten your vaginal muscles because you are already stretched. But then again, sometimes a man with an unusually large cock will be very good in bed, because he builds a woman up to the point of almost climaxing. The reason he does that is that he knows he will come immediately he starts fucking—because the friction is so tight. Really, though, I'd rather a man to not be too big or too wide, because medium to small men usually take more time in foreplay and make sure that I am ready. Men also worry about knowing if a woman has come or not. They don't realize that a woman isn't going to come every time she goes to bed. A man should be able to tell if a woman has come, by her reactions—my skin goes all sweaty, I get a red flush, and my breathing changes completely for several minutes.

Many men have their first sexual experience with a prostitute. How do you teach a virgin to have sex?

When I get a virgin I take the lead. I give him good head and then get on top and screw him. I do that so he gets the sensation and motions of screwing, without having to go through any awkwardness himself. The first time is strictly for the man's own pleasure—to release the tension from his system. The second time I teach him to explore me generally and teach him what it feels like to touch and hold a woman. Other men who are not virgins often want to learn how to eat a woman. Most men don't know that a woman's most sensitive part is her clitoris—that it turns her on or off. Some men can't even find it, or if they can they don't know how to treat it and just slubber and press instead of teasing it. A lot of guys think that eating a woman means screwing her with their tongue—which feels good once a woman is really turned on, but doesn't turn her on in the first place.

Some women I have talked to fantasize about "making" a hooker orgasm. What makes you orgasm?

I only come when I am eaten, but I need more than that. Straight screwing doesn't turn me on, mostly because of having to do it all the time when I am working. I like a man who lets me be lazy for a while so I don't have to do the work. In my work I always have to be forward, so I like it when the man takes the lead. I like a man who is very tender to me—doesn't push, doesn't jump on me, but rubs my back first and tries to relax me. I like a man who is very gentle, but also very much in control—who tries things, starts doing something to me, then watches my reactions to see whether I like it or not. Then he will back off if he feels I don't like something, or proceeds if he feels I do like it. A good lover pays attention to a woman's reactions and never tries to manipulate her into doing something she doesn't like. A lot of men may ask what pleases me, but I can soon tell they don't really care what pleases me—only that *they* come. The ideal man in bed—the kind that makes me come—relaxes me first, goes out of his way to please me, really *needs* for me to enjoy the sex, and only enjoys it if I do.

Harry Reems

A European duchess once told me she believed that the world is divided sexually between voyeurs and participants. Well, I don't much like porno movies, but I did see Harry Reems in *Deep Throat*, and once met him at a Beverly Hills

party. I arranged to interview Harry at his Malibu
Beach house and was parking the car when Harry
came out to take in the mail. My first impression
of Harry Reems was far from pornographic—do-
mestic, gentle, with tea-colored eyes and a droopy
Victorian mustache. Inside the beach house we sat
looking out at the Pacific, ate nuts out of a glass
jar, and talked. Before I left, I commented on
Harry reading *Whatever Happened to the Class of
'65?* and Harry, rather wistfully, said, "You know,
I also belonged to the class of '65."

Harry Reems must be the most famous porno
star in the world—and I naturally asked him how
he did what he does so often. For men who are
curious about his superstud techniques, he reveals
how he turns himself on at all times, how he holds
back from an orgasm, how he recognizes a
woman's orgasm (which he admits is difficult at
first), and how he discovers the sexuality of a new
woman.

In one day of filming, I have two sexual encounters
lasting anywhere from two to four hours. Sometimes I
have trouble getting an erection in front of the
cameras—generally because I'm tired from being out
the night before, or it may be late afternoon and I have
been making love for hours. So I stop for a while, then
start again. If I don't get it up again, we break for the
day, then pick up the scene the next day. But usually, I
guess, I can go on forever, for a long, long, long
period—for hours without having an orgasm.

I hold back from my orgasm by knowing that I'm
limited to just one. So when the sexual act is great,
with good sensations and feelings, and I don't want it
to end, I say to the woman, "Let's stop—don't let me
come—I don't want to yet." So I wait until the throbbing and pulsating of my penis subsides. I put my mind
into another sphere, another space, if I'm about to orgasm. If I'm enjoying the touch, the smell, the feel of

my partner, I simply avoid the sensation, I turn off my nose to the odors, and think about something as distant from the situation I am in as possible.

I don't think a man can easily recognize a woman's orgasms. I have women friends who are extremely violent and verbal in their orgasms—but then there are other women who orgasm in total silence. Although, if I am still inside a woman I can feel certain physical sensations, the vaginal contractions. Many women become extremely sensitive after an orgasm, and if we make love in a very physical way the woman may have a contraction of small orgasms after the major one. Eventually, though, there will be a moment when she says, "Stop, it is too sensitive and painful." Then I either change rhythm completely, or perform oral sex on the woman—which will bring her to another orgasm. I love to bring a woman to orgasm—probably out of a macho feeling of "I brought her to orgasm, isn't that great." But if bed becomes "You do me and I'll do you" or "You've had your orgasm, now it's my turn" I think you fail in terms of emotional communication.

I worry about the woman having an orgasm if I am with her for the first time because I want her to know that I am capable. If I find the woman attractive and want to see her more than once, I don't want her to emerge from the experience thinking all I did was seek my own satisfaction, that I have no ability and didn't understand that the woman also needed to fulfill herself. Women are becoming a lot more aggressive in their sexual attitudes and performances. They now demand their own satisfaction. They say things like "Will you rub my nipples?" or "Would you turn me over?—I like it better from behind than from the front." Women are now expressing their sexual needs and desires, and I like that very much. When you go to bed with a woman for the first time there is an added electricity. The first time in bed with a stranger is exciting, because after you get to know a woman, although you become compatible, the sex does become almost routine. I find it very exciting to be in bed with new women all the time. I am a very sexual person, and I think sex dominates my life. I like all women in bed— busty women, physical women, dominant women, childlike women, I like them all. When I have sex in films I get turned on by having sex with someone I don't know. I walk into the room, say good morning to the director, he says, "This is Mary Smith," I say, "Hello," we shake hands, and I know that in an hour we'll be in bed. The woman is a beautiful stranger, there's no marriage dance, no seduction, it is strictly the physical act of instinctive sex—that, to me, is a turn-on.

Usually, though, a man should be able to discover the sexuality of the woman he is about to go to bed with. I can judge if a woman's sexuality is limited by her attitudes; if she is set in her ways and opinions, I will know that in bed she is also unexperimental, inexperienced, and uncreative. If people are judgmental, if their creative expression is limited, then usually their sexuality is limited as well. If people experiment in their daily lives, are adventurous, then I think their sexuality is going to be stronger. But if they are locked into routines and are mechanized, I think their sexuality will be mechanical as well.

Once you're in bed with a woman you've got to find out what turns her on. I've been able to fulfill every fantasy I've ever had, and I discover the woman's fantasies by asking her. I experiment with her while we are having sex; I plunge my penis in really hard—in one thrust—to see if that excites the woman. I usually find that most women who are sensitive, soft, and sensual usually respond to a very physical act. Most women enjoy a good hard fuck. They really enjoy being fucked. I like to go in deep—but the man has to adjust his sexual rhythm to the woman's even if in doing so he loses satisfactions of his own. Every man has a sexual rhythm he likes best—you don't develop that, it's inherent. I see a lot of men fuck, and there is a difference in speed and depth. Some men will just put the tip in and go real fast on the outside. Other men will go in deeper, and when they get in deeper they push to go in even deeper and then pull out. Some men will push themselves in and when they are in they will push in farther without taking it out.

I like to see the woman reacting in bed. I like to see her performing. I am very visual—I like to look at the sex act to have lights on, to see the act that I am performing. I favor a position with the woman on her side, her legs folded up, not quite up to her chest, with the top of her torso turned up so she is facing up toward me—then I can see her react.

I am also experimenting with words right now. I used to think it was naughty and dirty to be very verbal in bed. I was afraid to act out the fantasy or use coarse language. Since then I have found that words excite me very much and in most cases also excite the woman. But with many women I don't talk in bed at all—it depends how compatible I feel with the woman before we go to bed.

Very few things shock me sexually, but I am shocked by extremes of sadomasochism. I like to make love from behind, in a doggy position; then, in many cases, I will start spanking the woman. If I find her reaction to the spanking is favorable, I will spank her a little harder. There are some women who want to make love in a very rough way, and it doesn't turn me on if the woman says "Harder, harder" till you get to the point where you're pulling her hair. A little spanking can be fun and exciting, but the excitement stops when the sex becomes brutal, induces pain, and is no longer really playing. I don't think you can give technical hints on how to be good in bed. The only way to be good in bed is to try to attain exactly what you want. If I had a son I would tell him that sex is a pleasurable exercise, a high form of communication. I would let him know that he will go through a period of frustration and fear at a young age but that it will all eventually work out for him. There are no rights and wrongs in sex—just whatever turns you on. If you want to be good in bed—if you want to be good at sex—practice it!

John Holmes

When I asked the late John Wayne what makes a woman good in bed, he replied, "Being there." I've never seen a John Holmes movie, but I do know that all he has to do is just be there—and display. Reputedly the best-endowed porno star in America, John Holmes was a complete surprise to me. First, because he maintains a Garboesque privacy, was nearly as difficult to find as Regine, never told me where I could contact him, so all arrangements were made through John's answering service, and we finally met at a secret address in Beverly Hills. I was also surprised because John Holmes seemed very shy and underplayed, was polite, with innocent blue eyes, curly blond hair, and college boy looks. I liked the way he understated his sexy image, and I found it ironic that John Holmes, who has what many American men most desire, doesn't use it much, and prefers to give a woman oral sex.

I've had ten thousand women. I've done over three thousand films—with an average of two girls a film—I went to orgies for two years—Fridays, Saturdays, and Sundays—then there were also freebies. A woman once paid me ten thousand dollars for a week of sex—we did everything imaginable.

How old were you when you first had sex?

I was eight when I started—I had a nursemaid and I was giving her very good head by the time I was nine. Daily. I looked forward to it. The nursemaid was twenty-three, she gave me baths, washed my genitals for a long time; I got a hard-on and one time just got off. Her room was connected to mine through a bathroom, and she would leave her door open so that I could watch her shower—she was a temptress.

What did she teach you about sex?

I had regular object lessons: "Get down between my legs—this is that—you touch this—stick it in." She gave me oral sex and told me how to avoid ejaculation. Most men are basically too fast—get too rapidly excited. You have to get that out of your system. You have to keep a hint of the animal—with the control of a human. I don't think I was born good—I think everybody is born bad, really terrible, and it's something you acquire. A man usually learns to fuck with a prostitute or during a nervous experience in the back of a car. But I was spoiled rotten—because I had regular sex for two years till I was ten.

What effect did being well endowed have on you while you were growing up?

I started getting teased by kids in the showers when I was in the third grade. I had a really good reputation in the school. I had girls run after me. If they were going steady with a guy they would break up just to go out with me for a weekend. It's good to get a reputation for being good in bed.

What was your sex life like during your teens?

Between the nursemaid and when I was seventeen I had sex whenever I could get it—not too easy for a ten-year-old. I lived in a bordello in Paris for a while—that's where I pulled my first trick. Bisexual women would come in and I would say, "How would you like a man instead of a woman?" and I'd go to bed with them. I developed oral sex in Paris, by doing it constantly. You only get good through experience, through constantly being in bed with someone.

How do you ask a woman to go to bed with you in noncommercial sex? The initial approach is very important and fifty percent of men don't seem to know how to make a sexy approach to women. What is your advice to all those men?

You have to get a woman alone, because every woman has a private personality and a public personality. It is also fifty percent body movement—contact and touch. It can be one three-second gesture—as the touch of a hand while lighting a cigarette, or the touch of a shoulder. Never grab a woman. If you grab a woman you are showing undisciplined or animal sex. That may be good when you're *in* bed, but for an approach it's terrible. Be gentle, be concerned, relax. You have to have a sexy look in your eye when you look at a woman. Never ask to go to bed with a woman—just imply it with decadence. Don't ever say, "I'd like to make love to you—I'd like to take you to bed." There are a million other lines. If you introduced me to ten women I could think up ten different lines. Lines like: "Do you like girls or guys or both?" "What is your favorite position?" "This is a most interesting party, but how would you like to come back to my place and check out my etchings?" "Do you know, I happen to give excellent head?" or "You know that you are beautiful—I would love to give you head—and I bet you'd love it."

I expected you to emphasize your size—instead you keep talking about head. Why is that?

I love to give head. I like to give a woman head and not even take my clothes off. Most men really like getting head—they give a woman head and then expect it in return. I don't—I would rather give head than get it.

What is your advice to the man who wants to be good at giving women oral sex?

Give it as you would like to have it done to yourself. Think of a woman's lips as testicles—they have the same feel. The clitoris is like the head of the penis—the only difference is that the woman has a vagina. Stimulate the lips—go down on the woman very slowly—pay close attention to her eyes—and plan on not climaxing yourself. Do it relaxed—do it slow. No harsh movements—slow, tender movements. Keep your breathing slow—if you're overanxious, if you're nervous and shaking, that is going to throw the woman off completely.

Many women I've spoken to worry about the time it takes them to orgasm. How long should a man expect to give a woman oral sex?

A man should expect to do it as long as he likes. I know girls who are wet when you go down on them and come in sixty seconds. Other women can take forty-five minutes—which doesn't matter as long as the woman is enjoying it. If she's enjoying it, stay down there—she'll let you know when to give up. I stop after fifteen to twenty minutes and have a cigarette or a drink when I am giving head.

A lot of men worry about recognizing a woman's orgasms—and we both know that women fake. So how do you think a man can tell if a woman has orgasmed?

If you're giving a woman oral sex you can taste her come. In fucking, if you cannot tell whether a woman has climaxed or not then she has generally not. But you don't always feel the contractions—some women climax interuterinally. But if you are performing head

on a woman and the woman is not generally enjoying
it, you ought to be able to tell. Then you have to look
the woman in the eye and say, "What am I not doing
right? What do you like? How do you like it? Am I not
hitting your clitoris rightly? How do you like it—faster
or slower or deeper?" If a woman won't communicate
with you sexually while you're making love to her, she
has got more sexual hangups than you should be
messing around with.

How do you discover a woman's sexual fantasies?

A woman will usually indicate her sexual fantasies
and preferences. If you touch her anus, for example,
and she tightens up, that is an indication that she
doesn't like anal sex. If she pushes her butt toward your
finger, then you can tell that she is into anal sex. If I
give a woman head and then stop and she pulls me on
top of her, I know she likes to fuck. Then you can tell
a lot by position. Many women like to be taken—without words, just animalistic, savage sex. Those women
respond best to the Syrian rape position. It's a very
friendly position which allows total touching of both
bodies, but the man also entraps the woman. She is on
her back and he is on his side—it is difficult to explain
in detail. I am rough with some women and gentle with
others.

Do you have very strong stamina?

No—I just like to make love. Getting a hard-on is
never a problem. I could have sex nine times a day. I
don't think about getting myself off—just about getting
the woman off. I constantly want to make the woman
climax. Not to the extent that she is exhausted. I've
had women go to sleep on me, I've had women pass
out on me, I've had women climax eight, nine times and
then act disinterested. Five or six orgasms is good. If
you make a woman climax more than her limit, she
won't give you a performance.

Is the man who is good in bed always ready to make love?

No. A man who is really good in bed and has a lot of women is very choosy. I go to bed with one out of ten women who want to go to bed with me. You can't have them all.

Do you ever feel pressured to perform in your private life?

No—if I feel pressured I just don't do it. I just say, "I've had a really bad day today—I don't want to fuck," or "I'm terribly tired—it will be a terrible performance." Women use excuses like that all the time. I am never pressured into being John C. Holmes. I am two different people—no one in this world can possibly be John C. Holmes. *I* can't be him—*he* is everything to everybody who wants to go to bed with him. I am John Holmes and I enjoy my sex—and when I am working I am John C. Holmes.

John C. Holmes is renowned for the size of his penis—what effect does that have on your private life?

I think women want to go to bed with me because of it. I have friends who love me because of my cock, because I know how to fuck, and just that. Then I have a lot of other friends whom I never go to bed with. Having a big cock is an image. Women like to stare at it—when I get an erection they just want to get in between my legs and touch it. A woman has never said that my cock has hurt her, because I do a lot of foreplay. But I have never yet had a woman who could swallow more than half my cock in oral sex.

How important is size in making you good in bed?

I have had women tell me that guys almost as big as me are bum fucks—premature ejaculators, or unable to get it up. Nervous. Having a big cock is nothing to do with it. It all depends on how many times you've done it and how much you know about women. A big cock just helps in *getting* women. If you are wealthy you are also going to have a lot of women. But if you are broke and have a little dick—find someone who can love you for what you are. Never try to be ten different people—never try to be the world's greatest lover. Don't push so much. If you want to make love to a woman, don't do it nervously—do it with the thought in mind that you are going to make love to her and make her climax. If you are nervous and ejaculate prematurely, give the woman head and forget about your own climax.

What is your advice to the "average" man who wants to be good in bed?

Treat the woman better than yourself. Be more attentive to her needs than to your own. Become good at what you like getting. Don't be rushed—sex is not a five-minute thing, sex is an all-evening thing. If you go to bed with a woman for five minutes she will feel worse than a whore. Be slow, be calm, think continually about the woman, don't think about yourself. Forget "me"—think "her." Talk to the woman. Women are human beings, but most men forget that and think of them as flesh-colored containers for come. Most men don't realize that all women are physically, mentally, and emotionally different and that they have to try to understand each individual woman. Sex is a smell, a taste, a flavor, skin, shapes of clitorises—no woman has the same shape clitoris. Be good with your mouth. Make love to the woman with your mouth. Your lips, the inside of your lips, your tongue. Everything is important, and if you can get a woman stimulated orally, then she will get off on your cock—no matter what size it is.

Have you ever felt sexually inadequate?

Men have got five million things to think about that women haven't. Women aren't pushed into a place in society where they are forced to make a living and support others. A man has the world on his shoulders, and sex is the third or fourth thought in his mind. But it is terribly important for a man to be good in bed. However, I think that if a man is not good in bed it may also be the woman's fault. When making love to an immense amount of women you find out that one woman out of ten is going to satisfy you mentally and physically. Every woman you go to bed with is not going to be great. Many times you would get more out of the experience by masturbating. I can be terrible with some women and can't satisfy them. That happens when a woman goes to bed with me because she wants a part in one of my films. When I find out I feel from her vibrations that she doesn't want to be in bed with me. Then I just say, "I know you're not going to enjoy this, so neither am I—let's quit."

How does being in love relate to your sexual performance?

Usually when I go to bed with a woman I like I can come six or seven times in an evening. But when I am in love with a woman I can only make love to her once a night, because it takes everything emotionally, mentally, and physically.

The last question has got to be about your claim to fame—has it ever been a disadvantage?

Yes, at orgies—because many times I've been the only man there who hasn't been allowed to make love to any woman he wants to. Husbands have forbidden their wives to have sex with me—any other man at the orgy, but not me. I don't get annoyed, though—there's nothing I can do about it. I am not a proud person—I am not an egoist. My thoughts are basically gentle. I create life the way I want to live it—I am just another guy and I only do just another job.

Tony

Tony is a Las Vegas male prostitute for women—but I couldn't imagine going to bed with him in a million years, because I wasn't turned on by his beefy redneck looks. Male prostitution for women is well organized in Las Vegas. The *Las Vegas Panorama* newspaper advertises "male escorts." The Las Vegas Police Department licenses the escort agencies, and each male prostitute is subject to regular medical inspections. Las Vegas male prostitutes charge women from $70 an hour, and also expect to be tipped. If a woman wants to buy a session with a male prostitute in Las Vegas, she calls the agency, asks for an escort, stressing that she wants to "stay at home" with him, and describes her type of man. I learned that the women who pay for sex are sometimes in their twenties, afraid to risk a pickup in crime-ridden Las Vegas. Other women want to buy sexual experimentation, unwilling to risk suggesting it to a man they love. Occasionally fathers pay male prostitutes to devirginize their daughters. Other customers are famous women, or wives of famous men, seeking sex plus discretion.

Although I believe that as long as men have the opportunity to pay for sex, women should have the same opportunity, Tony's interview highlights aspects of prostitution common to both sexes—dishonest flattery and faking enjoyment, which clients presumably want and pay for, the sad facets of prostitution. Here Tony tells how he does it, making it very clear that he is in prostitution for the money.

Being a hooker is an easy way for me to make money. When I signed on with the escort agency no questions were asked, no advice given, and I didn't have to take any kind of test. I don't have a fixed price—I try to get as much money as possible out of the women. The agency sets a fee for the evening, but it's up to me to charge what I like for the sex; I never go to bed with a woman for less than fifty dollars. Usually I get up to two hundred, but if the girl is ugly I charge three hundred. The other day I got five hundred from a couple—because the husband paid extra to watch while I fucked his wife, then gave her head afterwards.

The women I see are eighteen and up—last month I even had a broad of seventy. I couldn't get it up, so I called another guy to take over. I never know beforehand what a girl is going to look like. Sometimes I see really beautiful girls who want me to act out a fantasy they are ashamed to do with their boyfriends; I once had a fabulous-looking air hostess who wanted to be destroyed. Apparently everybody worshiped her and kept telling her that she was beautiful so that she had developed a need to be degraded. So I put clothespins on her body till she bled, pulled her hair, and marked her body—but only in the places that didn't show. I didn't get carried away—because I always control myself. Women I see often want to experiment, to do something different, like go to bed with me and a black stud, because they are paying and in Vegas no one will know what they have done.

Pleasure seekers pay for sex in Las Vegas. Women who are away from home and want to let their hair down. Some women are embarrassed to tell me what they want—so as soon as I walk into the room I say, "What can I do for you?" The woman usually says something like "I've never paid for sex before, this is the first time—I'm here for two days while my husband is away, I'm lonely and I want someone to be with." Most of the women I see want me to give them head—because their husbands refuse to. So that I usually end up giving them head, then having sex with them.

However ugly a woman is, she usually wants compliments—so I say things like "You've got beautiful hair"—even though she must know I'm faking, because she is paying. Even if the girl is a dog I still tell her she is beautiful, then try to get the sex over with really quickly. I never have problems getting a hard-on—I just turn myself on by pretending the girl is good-looking or by fantasizing I am with someone else.

Some of the clients go stiff when I have sex with them because they aren't that sexy—if they were they would be getting it for free. The wild ones that really go nuts make me better in bed. If the woman gets turned on, then so do I. Sometimes a client is nice, beautiful, *and* goes wild—then I have to think of something else, otherwise I will come too soon. If a client really turns me on the first time, I won't charge her as much the second time, but I'll never do it for free.

I'm a very good sexual lover. I first had sex at seventeen. In those days it was difficult to persuade a woman to have sex with you—you practically had to marry her. Now it's easier, and I've also got better since I've had a lot of women. I'm not super-looking, I don't have a super body, but none of that matters once you've got the girl horny. I've had girls say, "Your cock isn't more than eight inches long—my husband has got more than that." So I say, "Let's give it a try," because I know that when a woman is really turned on, the size of a man's cock really doesn't matter.

Most girls do want a guy who will last a long time, especially girls who like to screw. There's a girl in Vegas who can take on six guys and still doesn't come—so if a guy only lasts fifteen minutes with her she gets mad because she needs an hour. If I survive the first five minutes without coming I can go on for three hours. Female hookers will tell you the same about their clients—if a man doesn't come within the first five minutes he will take forever. Which is a drawback for female hookers, who want the experience to be over quickly. My clients want me to last a long time, and I've had stamina ever since I was a kid and a great deal of staying power. I'm a sports handicapper and I take my mind off coming by thinking of sports scores—football or baseball, depending on the season.

Most guys can't go fast *and* last for a long time. The fast stroke has always been my best, and I go like a machine gun. Going fast all the time that you are fucking a woman makes her come. I can usually tell if a woman has come by the way in which she grips me with her legs. But I am not always sure. If every man could tell when a woman was faking, all the female hookers in Vegas would go out of business.

The best way for a man to be good in bed is to have a lot of sex. The more you do it, the more you'll like it and the better you'll get. The most important thing about being good in bed is to make a girl feel that you really like sex. To get really emotional when you're giving her head. Pretend that you really like doing it—even if you don't—because if the woman thinks you're enjoying it, that will get her off. Think about satisfying the woman—not yourself. And most of all, if I really want to get tips from a woman and make sure she comes back, I tell her she was fantastic; if you want a woman to think you are good in bed, just tell her that she was.

Sterling

I met Sterling by recommendation. A friend one day announced that her marital sex life had been saved because of Sterling. Her husband had flown from New York to L.A. and had met Sterling on the plane. They discussed sex. Sterling explained techniques to the husband, which he put into practice that night, and, said my friend, revolutionized their sex life. As a beneficiary, she strongly advised that I interview Sterling, in an attempt to discover his secrets, and obtain sexual advice for other men.

Sterling is thirty-eight years old and black. He has been a male prostitute for twenty years. I interviewed him at his house in East Los Angeles—his three children were in the room, and we talked for two hours. Sterling was quiet, far removed from the black-superstud image too many movies project. Sterling works outside the framework of structured male prostitution, haunting Marina Del Rey bars, always alone.

I can make love to any woman that wants to be made love to. And I can make love ten to fifteen times a night. I used to give regular sex classes to my son when he was fourteen. I showed him how to maneuver his tongue—to work it backward and forward in his mouth, to push it against his teeth to strengthen the muscles. I told him to practice and build up the muscles in his tongue, train the tip so that it hardened and tingled—then he would have it made when he had sex with a woman. Even if my son doesn't become a male whore I want him to be good in bed.

I learned to be good in bed through practice—through making myself available to a variety of women who taught me. The first woman who taught me about sex was Ellie May—she was sixty and I was fifteen. When I would go to her house in Chicago she would walk around half-dressed. Then one day she had me lie down on the bed with her and said, "I'm going to teach you something that will help you get along in the world, how to give a woman oral sex." So she got me down there, I froze up, and she bribed me by giving me a present. Each time I froze up she would always bribe me—so that at first oral sex was just an obligation. I was also a little rough until Ellie told me, "I'm not supposed to feel your teeth, not too much suction, do it lightly and run your tongue backward and forward over the clitoris—slow and gentle."

Then I met the neighborhood tramp. I bet the guys that I could have sex with a girl just like they did, so I got into the back seat of a car with her, shaking like a leaf, wanting to do it right, but not knowing how. The sex was a great new experience—and I married the girl. After a while she was away for weeks with other men, and didn't even know if I was the father of her child. I wanted revenge on her and I decided never to be stuck on any one woman again. So I went to the Chicago Palmer House Hotel, sat by the pool, met an airline stewardess, and went to bed with her for sixty dollars. Then me and the bartender got tight and he introduced me to doctors' wives, judges' wives, and more airline stewardesses. All the women were white and never wanted anything from me but oral sex, because in those days white women didn't want a black man to climax in them.

Right now I've got eighteen women paying me—I make more money by working myself than by being a pimp. I don't have a fixed price, but I never go to bed for less than a hundred dollars. When I first started in California, though, it was different; I was working in a filling station and flirting with the women. One day a lady asked me what time I got off work. I told her I could get off that minute if she gave me thirty dollars. She paid me the money, I did it to her in the back of her car, and the next night she came back for more and brought her girlfriend. I screwed them both and they told their friends about me. Till it got to the point where I could afford to rent a room—where I went with a different woman every half hour. Nowadays I go to bars in the Marina or in Palos Verdes, where it's not hard to spot a lonesome woman. And it's lonesome women who pay for sex. I just roam, talk to the women, till one asks me what I do for a living. Then I tell her point-blank—I'm a male whore—so she can either take it or leave it. Women like that—they can have them for a night and never see them again.

Women have changed a lot since I started working. They enjoy sex more nowadays because they are not afraid to be demanding. It's very seldom that you get two women who like the same kind of sex. Many women still don't like to be really direct and say outright what they want in bed. Men should look for signs to help them discover what the woman wants. If the woman wants oral sex, she usually starts by having the man play with her breasts, then gradually puts her arms around him and pulls him down. If oral sex doesn't appeal to the woman, she will pull your head up, but she will rarely say, "I'm a square I don't like that"—she will just keep you away from that kind of position.

A man can tell if a woman wants gentle sex—because she will want to be hugged and pampered out of bed. But if a woman wants a man to be rough with her she usually starts with being rough with him. Her conversation is loud and fast and rude, she snatches, pulls, and wrestles with you. And when you get rough back she enjoys it in a resentful way—like rape. A man who is good in bed can be rough and gentle.

A man who is good in bed should help a woman experience things she has never tried before. If I want a woman to go down on me I don't say, "Hey, baby, why don't you give me a bit of head"—I just put myself in a position where she can get hold of it. Then she can take it or leave it. I don't ask her for anything. The night before last I was with a lady who didn't want her husband to give her head. He forced it on her—but I approached it differently. I played with her for a while, got her to the point where she thought I was going to climb on top of her and have intercourse, then I turned my body around to a position where my head was by her knees. She opened her legs, I started playing with her clitoris with my hand, and before she knew it I was playing with her clitoris with my tongue. She was experiencing something she had never had before, and it drove her wild; she didn't know what she was doing, but she came because she was exhausted.

Most of all I enjoy giving a woman oral sex. I enjoy seeing her go through the changes—then I know I've done my job well. I don't use vibrators or anything phony. If a woman wants vibrations I can give them to her with my tongue. I really like giving a woman oral sex until she can't take it anymore. That makes me feel good. I can do it to a woman for two hours—so that she has four or five climaxes. But usually after half an hour of oral sex a woman doesn't want any more, doesn't want to be penetrated. But I still like to have intercourse with a woman—otherwise she's only getting half of the sexual relationship.

I can tell by the slight trembling if a woman's climaxed. Then she relaxes, and if she's had a good climax she doesn't want you to move around, because every time you do, a certain nerve will make her jump. I've never had a woman fake an orgasm with me, but I've faked in bed. There are a lot of dumb women in the world who don't know when a man has climaxed. And I fake if I find one; make a lot of noise, grunt, squeeze the woman close to me, then relax and roll over. Then the woman thinks I've come.

As a professional I mustn't reach a climax before a lady is satisfied. I can have sex with a woman for one and a half hours or however long it takes her to reach real satisfaction. It's mind control. I turn off—I don't want to give up my pleasure to climax. If I get to a moment where I think I am nearly climaxing I change position and think of something else. I could look at a flowerpot, still enjoy the sex, but not reach a climax because I didn't want to. I just don't think about the sex. My penis is longer than average, but thin. Length satisfies every woman, length really matters, not thickness, because thickness is mostly at the top. Men who have fat penises usually can't go in deep. And if a woman wants it deep she doesn't want if off the top—she really *does* want it deep, and if you can't give it to her that way you will lose her. A man can recognize a woman who wants it deep because she will try to put her legs up over her head. But if a woman keeps her legs down she is usually tight and doesn't want the man to go deep because that will hurt her. You can always tell how a woman wants sex by the way in which she positions herself.

A man should follow the woman's rhythm, because she knows the best rhythm which will bring her to a climax. If a woman likes to go real slow and lazy, it means that she likes long-drawn-out sex acts. But if a woman is overheated she will also have a tendency to start going fast as soon as you put it in. She wants you to hurry up because she wants you to have the first climax quickly. Then if the man can hang in there he will really give the woman a big climax.

It helps a lot if the man moves the woman around in bed, maneuvers her with his hands. My hands are very soft, and when they sweat, they cool a woman's body. I have a very feminine, gentle touch, and when I touch a woman she feels my touch throughout her whole body, even if I only touch her with my fingertips. I take my time—a man who is good in bed is never in a hurry.

I never talk to a woman in bed—I find that when I talk to a woman in bed I lose what I am doing. I very seldom talk fantasies, unless they are asked for. Sometimes women do say, "Talk to me." Then it's hard for me to find things to say—and I rarely do say very much because I'm using all I've got.

I like anything in sex, except fat women. I can't perform with fat women and I never take money from them. It's a mental block. The oldest woman I've ever had was Ellie May, and the youngest was sixteen. She'd only ever been with older men, so I gave her what she'd never had; she always did for men, but they never did for her. When I gave her oral sex she went wild.

I've even paid whores who appealed to me—because there was no hassle involved. I find, though, that a black prostitute will jump into a car faster with a white man than with a black man. In general black women always yield faster to a white man than white women do to black men. It's in the blood of black girls to want white men—black mothers tell their daughters to get a white man who will do something for them. Black girls are told to "leave that nigger alone," so when a black man says, "Hey, baby," to a black girl she puts her nose up at him. But if a white man approaches the same girl she'll smile and say yes immediately. I think that inequality makes black men better in bed. A white man never has to prove anything sexually, while a black man constantly has to prove himself to a woman, and the need to prove himself is what makes a man good in bed.

Rick

I interviewed Rick on his own territory—a half-finished apartment in Greenwich Village. Rick sees men and women on alternate days; the day I interviewed him was, he told me, men. When I arrived, a muscleman was leaving; when I left, a thin boy arrived, with a pizza pie. Thinking of pizza pies, Rick says, makes him hold back from an orgasm. Rick looks like John Denver, with slight build and thick glasses.

Rick's interview covers almost every type of sex —homosexuality, heterosexuality, sadomasochism, and orgies—as well as general techniques for men. Like all the superstuds and hookers, Rick places paramount importance on giving a woman oral sex.

There is no difference in being good in bed with a man and being good in bed with a woman—you have to devote the same amount of emotion, care, and love to both sexes. I find sex with men and women equally satisfying. If I were told I could only have one more sexual experience in my entire life I would have an orgy with fifty men and fifty women. But if that experience had to be with one person only I would be unable to choose between being with a man or a woman—so I would masturbate instead.

Professionally I see men and women on alternate days. But nowadays I also see a lot of straight men professionally as well. Recently so much has been written about gay sex that straight men feel pressured to have sex with other men, and I often see basically straight men who feel the need to experiment with homosexuality. At the same time, many homosexuals I see, even now, still have problems in coping with the old taboos on having sex with other men. They are very uptight about their homosexuality, and some will only go to bed with another man if a woman is part of the scene. I try to overcome those prejudices, make the man feel very comfortable, spend a lot of time with him and try to be gentle and understanding.

It's astounding how many men are worried about penis size. I am hung very well—ten inches—but I never think of myself in terms of size or compare myself with other men. Yet I've had scenes with men who were bigger than me, but still thought they were small. Obviously my size can be a problem; some men are too tight and a few women are afraid to let me ball them because they think my size will hurt them. So I don't think that being big makes me better in bed—except that when both men and women see the size of my dick they fantasize about it.

Fantasies are very important to good sex; but you

can have a great fantasy partner who is not a good sex partner and vice-versa. In my private life I have two distinct fantasies I act out with men. I enjoy screwing great big muscular truck-driver-type men, or being screwed by very petite, very feminine, very obviously gay men. Today I wanted to be with very hot-looking muscular men—so I picked them up in the Village and so far I've already had six orgasms with different men. The women I fantasize about are either very sporty, healthy Farrah Fawcett types for fucking sex, or petite, feminine, pretty women for fantasy sex. I also like women of around forty-five.

The women I see professionally are mostly referred to me by their friends. I used to advertise as a male model in the "situations wanted" column of *The New York Times*. That column no longer exists, so I advertise in other New York papers. A woman calls me up and makes an appointment to see me. She arrives, we have coffee and a joint, then I interview her about her past sexual experiences and how far she wants to go. The price depends on what a woman's like and what she wants, but very often a woman knows what her friends have paid me and wants to compete with them by paying me more. Other women also tip.

There isn't a particular type of woman who will pay for sex. But mostly I see submissives who are into sado-masochism. Many of the masochistic women have status and power professionally, but want to be dominated in bed. Before I start I make sure the thresholds of the scene are verbalized. If the client wants to be beaten I ask if they are into pain. Some women want to be beaten with canes and belts and whips—so that they can then exhibit the marks to their husbands or lovers. I've also had dominant men pay me to be submissive. Mostly it's just spanking, but if things get too rough, I just stand up and end the scene.

I don't have any problems getting a woman into bed in my private life. In the '50s everything was different, full of proprieties. You waited before making a move, planned your seduction, and set up a dinner date. Then you had candlelight, mood music, good wine, and good marijuana. Then perhaps . . . Women today are much more sexually aggressive and suggest going back to my apartment themselves.

Some men still find it difficult to persuade a woman into bed. I think directness is most successful. I am very exhibitionistic about my body, go to the gym and take care of it. I play up my sexuality by the way I dress. A woman can often judge a man's sexuality by looking at his clothes; an aggressive dresser who wears layered looks, collarless shirts, and Cardin suits will usually be aggressive in bed. Whereas men who are more experimental with their clothes are also more sexually experimental. Many men who wear conservative clothes are usually conservative in bed. I dress in a very sexual way; I wear tapered shirts so the woman can see my chest, and tight trousers so she can see my ass and crotch. If I see that the woman is looking at my chest, I get myself into a position where she can touch it. Because that will arouse her. But I never *ask* a woman to go to bed with me—we just arrive at my apartment and I take my clothes off.

Some men have problems in verbalizing to women; in telling them what they want and finding out their fantasies. It's very difficult to discover a woman's fantasies before you go to bed with her; I always leave a copy of De Sade on my bedroom table—women flick through it and I judge their reaction, which is a great way of finding out what excites the woman. A man should definitely ask the woman what satisfies her. If he is nervous he ought to take half a Valium first, then ask her things like "Can I do this?" or "Would you like me to please you that way?" or "Have you ever thought of that?"

Then once he is in bed, a man should try a variety of things and should be able to pick up leads from the way in which the woman responds. For example, I fondle a woman's nipples, then say, "Do you want me to do that harder?"—because some women like to be manipulated quite roughly. If I see the roughness excites the woman, I carry on fondling her breasts with one hand, and with the other hold her arms above her head. If she enjoys that, then I know the woman will like some kind of restraint. Then I might put my feet on top of her so she can't move because my body has put her into basic bondage. At that point I might say, "Why don't you stop for a while and take a break?"

We stop, smoke a cigarette or a joint, which makes the woman realize that I am relaxed and not into just screwing. That will make her relax with me in a sexual way. Then I say, "Why don't we try something else? Why don't I tie your legs up." The woman's hands are still free, but having her legs tied creates eroticism. Then if that arouses her I hold her hands down so she is in total bondage.

Then I would probably go down on her. A lot of women love being eaten by a man but tell me that a lot of men still won't do it, which is surprising as it's so erotic. When I've eaten a woman for a while I stop and ask her if I'm doing it right—"Do you get off on my eating you?" I try and get her to respond verbally, because once you persuade a woman to open up verbally the fantasies will pour out of her. If she still doesn't tell me, then the next time I am with her I will try something different. Perhaps I will keep the lights on and make the woman look into the mirror while we are making love—so that she can watch her own femininity and grace. That will keep her connect visuality with safety and pleasure—and if a woman feels safe then she will also verbalize her fantasies and even act them out.

I was born good in bed, but I was always concerned with becoming better. I learned the techniques and details through experience. I had preliminary sex with girls when I was six. When I was eight I formed a sex club in my neighborhood where I had exploratory sex with three boys and a girl, and when I was nine I had proper sex with a girl. All I knew was that I had to touch the girl's breasts, get a response, then fuck her. Afterward I went to the library and read up on the anatomical background.

In my teens everything was refinement. I remember trying to unclasp a girl's bra from under her sweater. The bra got caught in the sweater, ruined the erotic atmosphere, but also taught me to take sweaters off first. Another time I was in bed with a girl and there was a party going on in the next room. Suddenly I had to go to the bathroom but didn't want to walk through the party with an erection. So I leaned out of the window and relieved myself that way, which also taught me always to go to the john before having sex.

Nowadays I can screw all night. I stop myself from coming by thinking of something other than sex. I think of pizza pies—if I imagine eating a fabulous pizza pie, then that takes my mind off sex. Or else I just stop for a break, get up, and do something else for a while. Techniques like that do help a man to be good in bed. But I think I am probably even better in bed when I love somebody, because then I become more trusting. I become more willing to experiment or try new positions or sex acts. My advice to men who want to be good in bed with most women is this: first take the phone off the hook, then think of the woman, then talk to her. Next think of yourself and try not to suppress your fantasies, then persuade the woman to tell you exactly what she *really* wants to feel.

SUMMARY OF
SEXUAL ADVICE AND TECHNIQUES

1. Care about the woman's orgasm.
2. Don't hold a woman's legs over her head.
3. Watch a woman's reactions to what you do and see if she likes it or not.
4. Never force a woman to do something she doesn't want.

5. Relax a woman before sex.
6. Hold back from an orgasm by stopping till the throbbing and pulsating have subsided.
7. Recognize the female orgasm by the woman's sensitivity after sex.
8. Try to discover a woman's sexuality by discovering her attitude to life.
9. Adjust your sexual rhythm to the woman's.
10. Practice sex.
11. Never grab a woman.
12. Be gentle and concerned, and relax.
13. Have a sexy look in your eyes when you look at a woman.
14. Never ask to go to bed with a woman—imply it with decadence.
15. Give the woman oral sex the way you would like to have it done yourself. Be slow and relaxed, with no harsh movements.
16. If the woman's not enjoying sex, ask why not.
17. Never try to be ten different people—don't try to be the world's greatest lover.
18. Be good at what you like getting.
19. Don't rush.
20. Talk to the woman.
21. If you are nervous, give the woman oral sex and forget about your own climax.
22. Make love to the woman with your mouth, your lips, the inside of your lips, your tongue.
23. Give a woman compliments.
24. Try not to orgasm during the first five minutes of sex. Then you will be able to go on for hours.
25. Go fast—then the woman will have an orgasm.
26. Hold back by thinking of football or baseball scores.
27. Make a woman feel you really like sex.
28. Get really emotional when you give a woman oral sex.
29. Tell the woman she is good in bed.

30. Push your tongue against your teeth to build up the muscles for oral sex.
31. You can tell if a woman wants gentle sex because she will want to be hugged and pampered out of bed.
32. If a woman wants rough sex she is usually rough with the man.
33. Help the woman experience new things.
34. Don't ask the woman to give you oral sex—just put her in the position where she can do it.
35. Hold back by not thinking of sex.
36. You can tell how a woman wants sex by the way in which she positions herself.
37. Follow the woman's rhythm, because she knows what makes her come.
38. Move a woman round in bed.
39. Persuade the woman to tell you exactly what she really wants to feel.

AFTERWORD
from Gore Vidal

Sex is both all the same and infinitely various. Until this generation, moralists could argue with complete conviction that the only acceptable sexual equation was "man plus woman equals baby." But now that half the world suffers from famine, that equation must be altered to: "man plus woman equals baby equals famine." To survive we must stop making babies at the current rate—and this can only be accomplished by breaking the stereotypes of woman the Breeder and man the Warrior. We must also realize that it is now no longer possible to maintain that sexual acts which do not create a child are unnatural—so it is no longer valid to say that certain sexual acts are "right" and others "wrong."

If we look back before the rise of Pauline Christianity we will see that sexuality was eclectic. The twelve Caesars were quite representative—except that their power enabled them to act out their sexual fantasies. The result encompassed anything and everything; given complete freedom to love, they went blithely from male to female as whim dictated—crisscrossing sexually without pattern or restriction. The Caesars demonstrated the wide variety of sensuality. They differed from their contemporaries only in that they had power.

Today twentieth-century man still considers heterosexuality as the norm. And most men today who have both sex and power generally prefer power. Power to them is the difference between major surgery and cosmetic surgery; major surgery is power, cosmetic surgery is creating a new character, while sex is just Band-aid. Power uses the psyche thoroughly—power is the completion of an ego that obviously has been wounded—otherwise it would not need the power. The powerful people I've known have been delighted by power, but tended not to be very much interested in sex. That doesn't mean they didn't have sex—just that it didn't prey on them, because power came first.

Europeans are more grown-up about sex than Americans because Europeans have fewer complexes, hence fewer obsessions. In America things are different because the country's Puritan founders (the Gores) combined with the Roman Catholic riff-raff of Europe; created Lyndon Johnson and *Penthouse*.

However, we are all a good deal less predictable and bland than anyone suspects. The only sexual norm is that there is no norm. What arouses X will repel Y—no two people react the same. So that any exploration of the extraordinary variety of human sexual response acts like those funhouse mirrors in showing us as we really are. And even though they may distort and mock the human figure, they never cease to reveal the real thing.

ABOUT THE AUTHOR

Wendy Leigh received her B.A. in English literature and the humanities from the University of Kent, Canterbury, England. She did extensive work in British radio and television as an investigative reporter and interviewer. She left the BBC to write WHAT MAKES A WOMAN G.I.B.* * GOOD IN BED, also available in Signet edition.

Recommended Reading from SIGNET

☐ **AN ANALYSIS OF HUMAN SEXUAL RESPONSE edited by Ruth and Edward Brecher.** A complete explanation for the layman of the controversial Masters-Johnson research on sexual response. Includes commentary by leaders in the study of sexual behavior, as well as prominent social critics.
(#J8440—$1.95)

☐ **AN ANALYSIS OF HUMAN SEXUAL INADEQUACY by Jhan and June Robbins.** A candid, accessible report on Masters and Johnson's Reproductive Biology Foundation. Described in layman's terms and clinical detail, here are the step-by-step techniques used by Masters and Johnson to help the sexually troubled achieve adequacy and physical fulfillment. Included are articles by Margaret Mead and Rollo May.
(#J8495—$1.95)

☐ **BEYOND THE MALE MYTH: What Women Want to Know About Men's Sexuality by Anthony Pietropinto, M.D., and Jacqueline Simenauer.** More revealing and comprehensive than THE HITE REPORT . . . "Fascinating . . . a landmark book . . . it's required reading!"—*Cosmopolitan*
(#E9040—$2.95)

☐ **LOVE WITHOUT FEAR by Eustace Chesser, M.D.** The classic sex manual by the foremost authority on love-making techniques. Filled with practical and scientific information, here is an explicit and plain treatment of the nature and need for intimacies between lovers, and a complete explanation of the methods of making the physical and psychological adjustments that are vital to a successful, mature relationship.
(#J8455—$1.95)

SIGNET Books You'll Want to Read

☐ **XAVIERA ON THE BEST PART OF A MAN by Xaviera Hollander.** Now the Happy Hooker lays it all on the line to share the joy of sex with you, recreating the lessons she's taught as well as the equally fascinating lessons she's learned in her intimate dealings with—THE BEST PART OF A MAN. (#E7848—$2.25)

☐ **XAVIERA'S SUPERSEX: Her Personal Techniques for Total Lovemaking by Xaviera Hollander.** An ultra-erotic tour through the world of sex by someone who has tried it all—every sensual possibility available to men and women of every sexual taste and level of expertise. A lavish, large-format bedside companion with 50 exquisitely erotic illustrations. (#E8384—$2.25)

☐ **HOW TO BE THE PERFECT LOVER by Graham Masterton.** Make love erotically—in ways you never thought of before. The book that tells you all you need to know to be the perfect lover. (#E8156—$1.75)

☐ **HOW TO DRIVE YOUR MAN WILD IN BED by Graham Masterton.** From the author of HOW TO BE THE PERFECT LOVER, exciting new erotic techniques to achieve the ultimate in sexual pleasure. (#J8744—$1.95)

☐ **THE POWER OF SEXUAL SURRENDER by Marie N. Robinson, M.D.** A whole continent of sensations and an emotional richness you never dared dream of await you in this enlightening book that offers hope to men and women who wish to achieve a mature and satisfying sexual relationship. (#W6921—$1.50)

Buy them at your local

bookstore or use coupon on

next page for ordering.

SIGNET Bestsellers You'll Enjoy